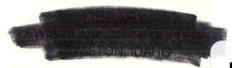

HEALTH AND INEQUALITY

How can research on the social determinants of health be translated into real-life public health practice? Challenging the research–practice gap, this text shows readers from a range of professions how their practice can help to minimise health inequalities. The social model of health embraces individual lifestyles, social and community networks, socio-economic, political and cultural influences and the plethora of factors that can impact on public health, for instance, education, work, welfare benefits, environment, housing, health and social care. All of these can have a significant effect on people's experiences of health and well-being, and are often unrecognised sources of health inequalities.

This innovative textbook outlines and discusses key public health principles and the social model of health. Drawing on a range of case studies and the international literature, it looks at how public health research has been applied to policy and practice. The book discusses the transferability that these findings have had and their capacity to influence and provide evidence for practice. *Health and Inequality* covers a broad range of social determinants of health, encountered throughout the life-course, including:

- pre-birth and early years
- breastfeeding and teenage mothers
- health inequalities for mothers and babies in prison
- children in full-time education
- sexuality, relationships and sexual health of young people
- early adulthood
- welfare rights and health benefits
- women, employment and well-being
- adults in later life.

Practical and clearly structured, this text will be useful to a range of health and social care professionals involved in public health work, particularly those undertaking courses on public health, health promotion or the social determinants of health.

Angela M. Tod is Professor in Health Services Research at Sheffield Hallam University, UK.

Julia Hirst is a Reader in Sociology and Public Health Lead at Sheffield Hallam University, UK.

This book brings to life the world of public health policy and practice. It provides tangible examples of how wider social determinants of health can impact on people's lives and ultimately prevent them from getting the care they need. This will be a valuable addition to every reading list for undergraduate and postgraduate courses concerned with health and wellbeing. It has a broad appeal across academic disciplines as well as health and social care professions.

—Linda Burke, Pro Vice Chancellor for the Faculty of Education and Health, University of Greenwich, UK

Julia Hirst and Angela Tod show that the strength of public health lies not only in the clinics and inside medical settings but crucially also in the societies in which people have to cope with systemic inequality and different access to care and support. With the rapid political and economic changes that so many societies are facing, public health needs are increasingly diverse and challenging. This book shows how public health and social care can be transformed and engages the reader in how theory and practice can combine and influence policy development. The range of topics covers most aspects of life and the eclectic mix of research is engaging and diverting and shows how public health can be effective and sustained.

—Mary Crewe, Director, Centre for the Study of AIDS, University of Pretoria, South Africa

HEALTH AND INEQUALITY

Applying public health research to policy and practice

Edited by Angela M. Tod and Julia Hirst

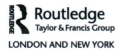

Routledge
Taylor & Francis Group

LONDON AND NEW YORK

First published 2014
by Routledge
2 Park Square, Milton Park, Abingdon, Oxon, OX14 4RN

and by Routledge
711 Third Avenue, New York, NY 10017

Routledge is an imprint of the Taylor & Francis Group, an informa business

British Library Cataloguing in Publication Data
A catalogue record for this book is available from the British Library

Library of Congress Cataloging-in-Publication Data
  Health and inequality (Tod)
  Health and inequality : applying public health research to policy and practice /
  [edited by] Angela M. Tod and Julia Hirst.
    p. ; cm.
  Includes bibliographical references.
  I. Tod, Angela M. (Angela Mary), editor of compilation.
  II. Hirst, Julia, editor of compilation. III. Title.
  [DNLM: 1. Health Status Disparities. 2. Health Policy.
  3. Health Services Research. 4. Public Health.
  5. Socioeconomic Factors. WA 300.1]
  RA440.85
  362.1072—dc23
  2013040328

ISBN: 978–0–415–63392–5 (hbk)
ISBN: 978–0–415–63393–2 (pbk)
ISBN: 978–0–203–09477–8 (ebk)

Typeset in Bembo
by Swales & Willis Ltd, Exeter, Devon

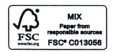

Printed and bound in Great Britain by
TJ International Ltd, Padstow, Cornwall

CONTENTS

ILLUSTRATIONS

Figures

Tables

CONTRIBUTORS

Katherine Albertson is a Research Fellow at the Hallam Centre for Community Justice at Sheffield Hallam University. She has eight years' experience as a qualitative researcher working across the criminal justice system. Katherine has specialised in developing empowering research methodologies with vulnerable cohorts whose voices are not traditionally heard, particularly offenders in custody.

Peter Allmark is a Principal Research Fellow in the Centre for Health and Social Care Research at Sheffield Hallam University. His health care background is in nursing; his academic background, in philosophy. In relation to public health, his interest is in how what is known about social determinants of health can be translated into measures that improve health whilst reducing health inequality.

Chris Bentley migrated from hospital medicine into population health via practice in East Africa, London, Sussex and South Yorkshire. He headed the Health Inequalities Nation Support Team for the Department of Health, and now works independently, with contracts at local, regional and national level, and with WHO in Europe. He has a Visiting Chair at Sheffield Hallam University.

Zoe Brownlie has worked with children, adolescents and families for twenty-five years. She currently works as a Clinical Psychologist for Sheffield Child and Adolescent Mental Health Service (CAMHS). She is involved in local strategic planning for early years emotional well-being and multi-agency training.

Catherine Burke was a Lecturer Practitioner Maternal and Infant Health and Care Theme, Yorkshire and Humber Health Innovation and Education Cluster (HIEC) at the Mother and Infant Research Unit at the University of York at the time of the study presented here. Catherine also has experience as a SureStart Midwifery team leader and as a Community Midwifery Educator. Catherine has since taken up a Senior Midwifery Lecturer post at Sheffield Hallam University.

Anna Clack is a Public Health Specialist at Rotherham Metropolitan Borough Council, where she is responsible for the management, delivery and evaluation of a range of public health programmes. She leads the Infant Mortality, Breastfeeding and Teenage Pregnancy agenda for Rotherham.

Eleanor Formby is a Senior Research Fellow at Sheffield Hallam University. Her research interests centre on lesbian, gay, bisexual and trans (LGBT) well-being, and on young people's learning about sex and sexualities. Currently she is conducting work regionally and internationally on homophobic and transphobic bullying.

Linda Grant is a Senior Lecturer in Social Policy. Linda lectures on policy, applied social science and public health. Her research expertise lies in how labour market and economic changes influence the lives of working-age women. Linda has worked on major European research collaborations on this topic. She has recently focused on women's part-time employment and the circumstances of women becoming disconnected from the labour market.

Julia Hirst is a Reader in Sociology and Public Health Hub Lead at Sheffield Hallam University. Julia's expertise lies in education and research on sexualities and sexual health with a particular focus on young people. She has an international reputation in her research field and has disseminated her work widely including lecture tours of New Zealand and South Africa. Julia's recent work explores how positive sexual identities and practices might be best promoted in school settings.

Georgina Lessing-Turner was, at the time of the study presented here, the Assistant Director of the Maternal and Infant Health and Care theme at the Yorkshire and the Humber Health Innovation and Education Cluster at the Mother and Infant Research Unit, University of York. Georgina has since taken a post as a Senior Lecturer in Midwifery at Edge Hill University in West Lancashire. Georgina retains a keen interest in midwifery supervision, advancing practice, and sustainability of change, leadership and organisational development.

Caroline O'Keeffe is a Senior Research Fellow at the Hallam Centre for Community Justice at Sheffield Hallam University. She has fifteen years' experience across many sectors of the criminal justice system, specialising in issues facing female offenders and qualitative methodologies.

Ray Poll is a Nurse Consultant for Viral Hepatitis at Sheffield Teaching Hospitals NHS Foundation Trust. He is nurse member of the Department of Health Advisory Group on Hepatitis. Ray is in the final year of the Doctorate of Professional Studies programme at Sheffield Hallam University. His research interest is in non-attendance at drug service hepatitis C outreach clinics: the experience of patients and staff.

Nick Pollard is a Senior Lecturer in Occupational Therapy at Sheffield Hallam University. He has a background in mental health, specialising in severe and enduring mental illness. His research interests concern community-based rehabilitation, community writing and publishing and political interpretations of human occupation.

Lindsey Reece is a Senior Researcher at the Centre for Sport and Exercise Science at Sheffield Hallam University. She has over ten years' experience of applied practice and research in public health. Lindsey's research focuses on designing and evaluating interventions to manage and prevent obesity across the lifespan.

Mary Renfrew, at the time of the study presented here, was a Professor of Mother and Infant Health and Director of the Mother and Infant Research Unit at the University of York. Mary has recently been appointed as Professor of Mother and Infant Health at the University of Dundee's College of Medicine, Dentistry and Nursing, where she is establishing a multidisciplinary programme of work on tackling inequalities in maternal and infant health and early years.

Angela M. Tod became committed to research and evaluation of health care and inequalities following an early career in cardiac nursing. She is Professor of Health Services Research at Sheffield Hallam University. She has over fifteen years' experience in research specialising in qualitative methods. Her research focus is on patient and public experience of health and health services, including factors influencing access to care. Her work is widely published and covers areas as diverse as lung cancer diagnosis, heart disease service access, obesity prevention and care, and fuel poverty and health.

FOREWORD

Public health, as a discipline, as a profession, as a 'science and an art', has rarely felt more challenging. Life expectancy has risen, but more years are actually lived with disability. We have longer lives, but not necessarily, it would seem, better health.

The biggest causes of premature mortality in the UK are still the same ones that were killing most people twenty years ago: ischaemic heart disease, lung cancer, stroke; and yet we have known for decades how to prevent these diseases. In the UK, we have introduced world-leading public health measures; we have made huge strides in cutting mortality rates from ischaemic heart disease. And yet our record on premature mortality still lags behind that of Europe. The enormous burden of disease attributable to tobacco may finally be waning but the epidemic of obesity is rising, with unknown consequences for the health of future generations.

This is the scale of the epidemiological challenge that is described in the Global Burden of Disease Study. Armed with this invaluable data, the public health community now has a much better idea of where it needs to focus its efforts and what it should prioritise in order to have the maximum impact on population health. What the data cannot tell us, however, is why we face the public health challenges we do, nor can they tell us how to apply what we know so that we improve health outcomes for all.

For that, we must turn to the ground-breaking work of Professor Sir Michael Marmot and his colleagues. The resulting conceptual framework, with its emphasis on the wider determinants of health and its life course approach, has profoundly shaped the way we think about and practise public health. It is fitting, therefore, that this framework should run as a thread through this book, which reflects on the way forward for public health.

To be involved in public health is to be concerned with the broader context of homes and jobs, of communities and surroundings, and how these influences play out at different stages of people's lives: from those foundational early years, through education, early adulthood, the working years and into retirement age.

To work in public health is also to recognise that the people who will make a difference to the wellbeing of children, families, employees and older people are not just health and social care practitioners but all those other dedicated professionals, ranging from teachers to community leaders.

The research and evaluation that is highlighted in this book, and its practical application throughout the life course, will undoubtedly be of relevance to this wider group of stakeholders as they collaborate in new ways to improve population health.

Indeed, this book could not come at a more opportune time: a time of momentous change as public health becomes the responsibility of local authorities. These are the natural leaders of public health because they are ideally placed to take action on the wider determinants of health. They have powerful levers to pull – across key sectors that we know influence health, such as housing, education, the local environment – and they understand their communities and their circumstances.

Those at the coalface, charged with translating this new era of opportunity into effective policies, will need practical support. They will find much to encourage and inspire them in these chapters, whether their priority is supporting families, young adults or older citizens. The hope is that we can reduce the gap between research and practice so that effective interventions can be implemented at scale, at speed and for the long-term. For the truth is that we cannot afford to wait decades to alter the course of this generation's epidemic of non-communicable diseases. The great public health pioneers of previous centuries combined pragmatism and great vision as they sought to transform the living conditions and life prospects of their communities. We need to apply these same values to tackle the preventable – and unacceptable – burden of preventable disease and disability that often falls hardest on the most vulnerable.

Professor Kevin Fenton
National Director Health and Wellbeing

ACKNOWLEDGEMENTS

This book was only possible because of the contribution of the chapter authors, to whom we owe a huge debt of gratitude. They have been committed to the ideas underpinning the book and diligent in the delivery of their work. Their generosity in sharing their ideas and work is appreciated. We hope that those who have participated have enjoyed the debate and discussion that has been generated along the way.

Special thanks goes to Chris Bentley, whose contribution to the content and process of delivering this book has been vast. He has contributed valuable reflections based on his unique experience, knowledge and insight in terms of the book chapters. Moreover he has guided and questioned discussion on core concepts and ideas proposed by all contributors, which has been both enjoyable and challenging.

We are also grateful to Rea Smith and Bronwen Moss who helped with the formatting of the original manuscript.

Finally, we would like to remember the contribution of the participants who took part in the research presented here. The insight that was generated was dependent on the participants sharing their time and experience, for which we are extremely appreciative.

1

PUBLIC HEALTH FOR A FAIRER SOCIETY

Angela M. Tod and Julia Hirst

Introduction

This is the first of two introductory chapters that present the landscape for public health and establish the context for this book. Each chapter is underpinned by a critical understanding of public health in various settings. Our broad priorities to address inequalities in health, fairness and social justice are best served by the principles enshrined in the *social model of health* (Dahlgren and Whitehead 1991a, 1991b, 2007), as this model has emerged as a legitimate vehicle for understanding public health policy and practice in the real world.

Chapter 1 considers the massive health divide in the UK and how public health measures have sought to address this. Its starting point is the Black Report (DHSS 1980), as this was the first evidence to highlight variations in health and mortality between population groups. We then describe how public health policy and practice changed in subsequent years, outlining policy aspirations and theoretical underpinnings in relation to core concepts such as fairness, social justice power and social control. The risk and reality of intervention generated inequalities will also be highlighted and discussed.

At the core of this book is an acceptance of the challenge laid down by the Leeds Declaration in 1993 (Long 1997). The Declaration took a radically new approach to developing public health evidence, based on wider socio-economic influences rather than biomedicine. The book aims to consider diverse approaches that can be adopted in research and evaluation and which aim to take up this challenge, reflecting the complex, multi-dimensional, multi-causal 'ecology of health' (Hunter 1994: Long 1993).

Understanding health

To establish the ideological and theoretical orientation of this book, we firstly explore what public health is, its definition, and locate the text within a social model of health.

- There is an urgent need to re-focus upstream, to move away from focusing predominently upon individual risks towards the social structures and processes within which ill-health originates.
- Research is needed to explore the factors which keep some people healthy despite their living in the most adverse circumstances.
- Lay people are experts and experts are lay people – lay knowledge about health needs, health service priorities and health outcomes should be central to public health research.
- The experimental model is an inadequate gold standard for guiding research into public health problems.
- A plurality of methods is required to address the multiple dimensions of public health problems.
- Not all health data can be represented in numbers – qualitative data have an important role to play in health research.
- There is nothing inherently 'soft' about qualitative methods or 'hard' about quantitative methods – both require rigorous application in appropriate contexts and hard thinking about difficult problems.
- An openness to the value of different methods means an openness to the contribution of a variety of disciplines.
- Public health problems will only be solved through a commitment to the application of research findings to policy and practice.
- Research funding should address the new directions that follow from these principles.

FIGURE 1.1   The Leeds Declaration: principles for action.

Source: Long 1993.

What is public health?

Agreeing a definition of public health has been a matter of much discussion and controversy. A commonly cited definition from the UK's Faculty of Public Health (FPH, the UK standards body for the public health workforce) masks some complex notions and values:

> Public health is 'the science and art of promoting and protecting health and wellbeing, preventing ill-health and prolonging life through the organised efforts of society'.
>
> *(FPH 2013)*

One complexity lies in recognising that public health is population-based, preventative in nature and focuses on promoting health and wellbeing in order to prevent ill health (Nuffield Council on Bioethics 2007). The focus is not exclusively on illness itself, nor on individuals, creating a dilemma for public health regarding which population to focus on. Taking a 'high–risk' population approach would require identifying people meeting specific risk criteria and targeting public health interventions at that sub-group. Where risk is spread across populations, a whole population approach may be more appropriate. An illustrative comparison is drug therapy strategies in high risk populations (e.g. statins in heart disease prevention), compared to legislation on salt, fat and trans-fat content, with the latter having been enforced in other countries such as Denmark, but not in the UK (Jones 2012). Some public health theorists such as Rose (1992) emphasise that most public health impacts can be derived from whole population approaches. Political motivations have prevented UK governments embracing such action, thus avoiding allegations of being 'a nanny state'. High risk population approaches have therefore dominated UK public health strategy and complex, commercial and legislative controversies linked to whole population interventions have been avoided.

A second complexity is that public health is integral to the way society works, its laws, politics and cultural norms (Rose 1985, 1992). The way society is organised will influence how people perceive health risk and health behaviour and influence their ability to follow public health advice. A common example is asking someone to stop smoking in a community where smoking is the norm.

A third challenge is that collective effort is required from all parts of society for public health. Success and sustainability are achieved not just by concentrating on individual lifestyle, but from the contribution of policy, planners, industries, education, health services, health professionals and lay people. For example, any success in addressing and preventing fuel poverty lies in partnerships between health, local government, housing, energy, education and voluntary agencies (see Chapter 17), as well as the people who are the target of public health interventions.

Finally, social justice is the foundation of public health as understood in this text. Whilst market justice proposes that entitlement (e.g. health and wealth) lies with the individual, social justice accepts that all people have basic entitlements such as health protection and a minimum income (Beauchamp 1976). Without these, the powerful influence of the environment, heredity or social structure will create health and financial inequalities.

The Faculty of Public Health does highlight principles of equity, empowerment, fairness, inclusivity and social justice as being central to public health:

> . . . a commitment to social justice lies at the heart of public health. This commitment is to the advancement of human well-being. It aims to lift up the systematically disadvantaged and in so doing further advance the common good by showing equal respect to all individuals and groups who make up the community. Justice in public health is purposeful, positivistic and humanistic. The aims of public health deserve a great deal more societal attention and resources than the political community has allowed.
>
> *(Gostin and Powers 2006: 1060)*

The decision to adopt a social justice model decision will influence the ethical and political framework for public health, and how the relationship and responsibilities of the state relate to the individual (Nuffield Council on Bioethics 2007).

A biomedical or social model of health?

In this section we critique the *biomedical* or *individual model of health* and summarise the key tenets of the *social model of health*. The latter evolved in response to the biomedical model and is established at the core of this book.

The biomedical model of health

A biomedical model of health is most likely to be applied in traditional Western health care and focuses attention on the individual, illness, diagnosis, prognosis, treatment and 'cure'. The biomedical model therefore lends itself to a 'downstream' focus and treats individuals who are ill, rather than taking preventative action (McKinlay 1975). It is argued that an 'upstream' focus would have more impact on population health; for example, proposing that legislative and fiscal measures to reduce tobacco consumption would prevent expensive 'downstream' biomedical intervention to treat smoking related ill health (McKinlay 1975; McKinlay and Marceau 2000).

Critics of a biomedical orientation (Blaxter 2004; Busfield 2000) argue that the biomedical model views the human body as little more than a machine, a 'thing' to be repaired when faulty. It does not take into account the broader influences on health and health related behaviour. Despite considerable criticism, the biomedical model remains politically prevalent in some contexts, particularly those underpinned by the ideological response of neo-liberals and the New Right to the free market and private medicine (for example see Navarro 2008; Resnick 2007; Wiley et al. 2013). Examples include the UK Thatcher government (1979–1990) and the Reagan administration in the US (1981–1989) where personal responsibility for health was emphasised in policy.

The social model of health

A social model of health does not negate the influence of age, sex, genetics, constitution and individual lifestyle factors, but sees health, illness and disease as integral products of the person/environment relationship (see Figure 1.2). In effect, this model emphasises social and economic influences and contextualises behaviours, health and illness experiences in relation to the everyday realities of people's lives. As Marmot (2010) has subsequently gone on to emphasise, the social model addresses all stages of the health/illness continuum and the dynamics of this throughout the life course.

By adopting a social model of public health, the primary concern of researchers and practitioners is to understand, explain and consider the influence of factors external to the individual. These are the social determinants, which are mapped out through the broader social, environmental and economic influences and that may be either protective of an individual or place them at risk of poor health (Dahlgren and Whitehead 2007). These determinants have varying significance for individuals and groups, in different contexts/places and at different times throughout the life course, but in broad terms it acknowledges that individual lifestyle factors are embedded in social, living and working conditions, and in community and wider socio-economic influences.

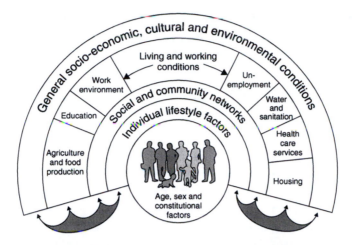

FIGURE 1.2   The main determinants of health (in Dahlgren and Whitehead 2007).

These factors are underscored further by mediators of health which we draw on throughout the ensuing chapters. These mediators or structural determinants include race and ethnicity, social class, gender, sexuality, age, socio–cultural factors, and place and space. These factors are significant to the experience of health and illness as well as access, uptake and experience of health care and social support. They became the basis of a *New Public Health* approach that developed in the 1980s, an approach that also placed new credence on 'upstream' preventative population based strategies.

Health inequalities: evidence and explanations for 'the health divide'

A brief overview of recent public health policy is presented here to provide the context in relation to health inequalities, alongside key evidence.

Health inequalities and public health policy

As stated, our starting point to describe the public health policy and practice context is the release of the Black Report in 1980 (DHSS 1980). Douglas Black was the first to collect substantial evidence that highlighted the salience of social class, gender and ethnicity to health inequalities (Black 1982; DHSS 1980). However, his report was preceded by 140 years of concern with socio–economic differentials in death rates (Macintyre 1997). Although Black's report displayed evidence of widespread health inequalities, the report publication was initially limited (on release, only 260 copies were made available over a Bank Holiday weekend), an action suggested to be politically motivated by the Thatcher (Conservative) government which resisted recognition of the extent or importance of the inequalities identified in the book.

Townsend et al. (1990) reanalysed Black's data and substantiated his conclusions. Margaret Whitehead (1987) also confirmed a 'health divide' as a trend of widening health inequalities. These reports found that health inequalities prevalent prior to the creation of the NHS in 1948 had not decreased, but were increasing with a growing class gradient in all major disease categorisations. Although Black emphasised that inequalities in health were directly affected by ethnicity, gender and social class, he emphasised the significance of occupational class and income. The influence of occupational class on health was further demonstrated in the seminal work of Marmot and colleagues in the Whitehall II Study (Ferrie et al. 2004) that provided unique insights into health inequalities.

The work of Black, Townsend and Whitehead fell on stony ground politically. The concurrent policy was influenced by market led, neo-liberal political economic thinking and resisted discussions about health inequalities and wider social determinants and influences. Western governments spoke euphemistically about 'health variations'. UK health policy emphasised the responsibility of the individual in maintaining healthy lifestyles and shied away from broader population based, upstream action and interventions. (Department of Health 1992).

In 1997, the elected New Labour government promised a different approach. Their White Paper 'Saving Lives: Our Healthier Nation' (Department of Health 1999) explicitly aimed to improve the health of everyone, but especially the poorest in society. It aimed to improve health and reduce inequalities through the mixed economy of care. The Acheson Report (1998) confirmed that inequalities relating to social class, gender and ethnicity persisted and that the explanations offered in previous reports maintained currency. Public health policy after 2002 was also heavily influenced by the reports of Wanless (2002, 2004), which outlined the resource implications for health provision, and which favoured a balanced up- and downstream orientation by tackling illness prevention as well as offering treatment and care.

Wanless (2004) also identified that the most disadvantaged in society experienced inequalities in accessing health interventions, along with a lack of understanding of the reasons for this. This gap in knowledge echoes the challenge set down by the Leeds Declaration of 1993. A number of health inequalities targets were identified in 2004, with the primary target being to reduce health inequalities by 10 per cent by 2010 and measured by infant mortality and life expectancy at birth (Department of Health 2009).

The Labour government and their subsequent policy was criticised for a focus on downstream health provision and individual lifestyle and behaviour (Crowley and Hunter 2005).

> Those working in public health should be encouraged to devote their energies to improving the health prospects for many minority groups within society whose health experience, and experience of health services, have been unsatisfactory and inexcusable in a civilised society . . . if we are to create the conditions in which the health of individuals and communities can flourish, action is needed on a whole range of social issues that determine the likelihood that a person will lead a long and healthy life.
>
> *(Crowley and Hunter 2005: 265)*

Public health policy was also critiqued for prompting interventions that aimed to reduce inequalities, but in reality made them worse. Such 'intervention generated inequalities' (IGIs) arise because the interventions disproportionately benefit less disadvantaged groups. It is suggested that downstream interventions, such as those that emerged from the policy 'Choosing Health' (Department of Health 2004), are more likely to increase inequalities than upstream, preventative strategies (Lorenc et al. 2012). For example, argument suggests that a national media or social marketing campaign promoting smoking cessation is more likely to increase inequalities than upstream fiscal, legislative or resource interventions such as tobacco pricing and the public smoking ban.

In the light of persistent and 'stubborn' health inequalities, a public health commission (Marmot 2010) was tasked with proposing evidence based policies and interventions that would strategically tackle the social determinants of health in the UK. Chapter 2 of this book addresses the Marmot Report in detail. Although commissioned by New Labour, the report had all-party endorsement and was released prior to the election of the Coalition government in 2010. A key theme within the report is that good health at birth and in the early years is a prerequisite to avoiding later health inequalities. Further, many of the factors that influence the gradient of health and inequalities relate to issues of social justice.

Evidence explaining health inequalities

Intrinsic to Marmot is a wealth of evidence that highlights factors influencing health inequalities. Some of these factors are summarised below, with reference to seminal evidence.

Materialist/socio economic factors are key to determining health status. They mean that those living with poverty are more likely to die younger and have increased illness throughout life (Black 1980). Wilkinson and Pickett (2009) argue that it is relative rather than absolute poverty that can have the most severe impact on health inequalities. He presents evidence to illustrate how disadvantaged communities in developed and Western societies have consistently widening health outcomes, despite policy interventions.

Women and girls are particularly affected, highlighting the influence of *gender* on inequalities. Globally, women experience greater poverty and less autonomy, resulting in dependency on a partner or the state (Benzeval et al. 1995). They are over-represented in poorly paid low status jobs (see Chapter 14) and those receiving benefits (see Chapter 13) are more likely to carry responsibility for unpaid caring and domestic labour (Doyal 1995). This renders women (especially those in ethnic minorities and lower social classes, and disabled women) with less access to material resources.

Scambler (2008) and Nazroo (1997) also argue that racial inequality ensures economic and environmental disadvantage for a majority of ethnic minorities. Evidence highlighting *race and ethnic* inequalities is problematic because it is inconclusive and not adequately representative of the diversity of ethnic groups; ethnicity is also influenced by socio-economic position, gender and place, hence it is difficult to distinguish variables. Having said this, numerous studies (Acheson 1998; Nazroo 1997; Scambler 1997) have found markedly different mortality and morbidity patterns between migrant and non-migrant populations. In summary:

> Not only do ethnic minorities suffer the general problems that reflect their class position, but they experience additional difficulties because of language and cultural differences or because of racial discrimination.
>
> *(Abercrombie et al. 1994: 401)*

Cultural/behavioural influences explain early deaths and morbidity among vulnerable populations. Individual and biographical behaviours and lifestyles also determine health (e.g. smoking) but our position here is that the latter should not be separated from socio-cultural mediators of health (Graham 2007). As indicated above, by critiquing core UK public health policy documents over the last 20 years, we can see the different perspectives regarding the role and responsibility of the individual in adopting healthy behaviours.

The influence of *place and environment* has also been considered in understanding and tackling health inequalities in global and local contexts. Globally, the average life expectancy at birth is 70 years (WHO 2011). However, rates vary enormously, with people in Mozambique, Swaziland, Zambia and Afghanistan having a life expectancy of 39–43 years, while those in Israel, Switzerland, Hong Kong and Japan live on average to 82 years. Across the UK, health gradients exist in relation to location, with the south-east of England experiencing better health and longevity than people living in parts of northern England, Scotland and south Wales (Dorling 2011). At a more local level, a health divide is evident within cities. Place and environment related health inequalities are closely tied to income, status, housing and housing 'churn' (Phillipson 2007; Wilkinson and Pickett 2009). Neighbourhood environments can impact on health outcomes and a subjective sense of wellbeing (Department of Health 2011: 57, Popay et al. 2003a, 2003b). For instance, lower income groups bear the disproportionate effects of environmental pollution (Dorling 2010). This can lead to the existence of food and service 'deserts' (Larsen and Gilliland 2008) with the most detrimental impact on those relying on public transport (Popay et al. 2003a, 2003b).

Finally, the influence of *age* as an explanation for health inequality needs to be considered. With biological age comes an increased vulnerability and risk of physical frailty, social isolation and consequentially, mental illness and mood disorders. However, it is not just biological deterioration that puts older people at risk. Wider social structures and systems may further compromise an older person's ability to be resilient, active and healthy (see Chapter 17). In addition, assumptions about older people and related stigma can reduce their ability to respond to public health messages (Day and Hitchings 2011; Hitchings and Day 2011), whilst inequalities can be further exacerbated by legislative measures, for example retirement or pensions policies.

So far in this Chapter we have recognised the importance of a social model of health in understanding health inequalities. A summary of health policy has been provided, bookended by Black (1980) and Marmot (2010). A brief overview of the factors influencing health inequalities has also been given. We now turn to the research agenda and associated challenges.

Understanding health inequalities research

This book aims to give voice to some public health research that provides insight into the real lives of people at risk of, or currently experiencing, health inequalities. In doing so, we hope to embrace the challenge of the Leeds Declaration. The methods chosen are diverse and the sample sizes vary enormously. Some of these studies are very small scale, examine local contexts and are focused on specific sub-groups. For this reason they may not normally be published or formally contribute to an evidence base. However, we believe that all the research presented here has value in providing understanding of why health inequalities arise and flag up considerations for public health policy and practice. This is illustrated in Table 1.1, where the chapter topics and methodologies are matched against outcomes in *Fair Society: Healthy Lives* (Marmot Review Team 2010).

Some small studies demand caution when claiming transferability and generalisation of findings; for example, a case study of two people (see Pollard, Chapter 16). However, they may provide a voice to people who would not be able to participate, or would not be invited to take part in more conventional experimental or large scale observational studies. Nor would methodologies such as the randomised controlled trial, that are placed higher in the evidence based medicine framework, be appropriate to examining the social nuances or the subtleties of upstream influences that people encounter during their lives and that make then vulnerable. A case is made for the complementary role of small scale and qualitative methodologies, alongside large experimental studies, within the public health research repertoire.

The complex public health landscape outlined above raises important questions regarding research and evidence, reflected in the Leeds Declaration. This is particularly true in contexts where professional voices are privileged, and policy development depends largely on data collected by GPs and other health professionals. Research questions include: Whose voices do we capture? Which data are valid and credible? Which data can we trust?

These questions relate to the type of research and evaluation we prioritise and fund. Since the Leeds Declaration, there has been a slow but notable shift in emphasis from an agenda that privileged the views of medical and scientific professionals and relied on epidemiology, randomised controlled trials (RCTs) and quantitative research, to one that recognises the value of the lay perspective and qualitative methodologies. To hear words, meanings, perceptions, feelings and experiences through qualitative research we enrich data provided by epidemiological studies. All too often this type of data is poorly funded and can remain in 'grey' literature that is not easily accessible. Thus, the evidence gets missed in scientific reviews of evidence and the 'voice' of the lay person remains hidden. Some of the work showcased in this text aims to capture the voices of people vulnerable to poor health and health inequalities. In doing so, the research recognises the importance of 'lay epidemiology' (Allmark and Tod 2006) which seeks to understand and give meaning to the values, knowledge, attitudes and beliefs of the public and how these influence health and health related behaviour and decision making.

In the following chapters you will find diverse methodological approaches adopted to answer public health research questions. It is our premise that they all, via different

TABLE 1.1 Chapter content, methodology and Marmot Objectives

Research Chapter/Methods	Marmot Objective 1 Give every child the best start in life	Marmot Objective 2 Enable all children, young people and adults to maximise their capabilities and have control over their lives	Marmot Objective 3 Create fair employment and good work for all	Marmot Objective 4 Ensure healthy standard of living for all	Marmot Objective 5 Create and develop healthy and sustainable places and communities	Marmot Objective 6 Strengthen the role and impact of ill health prevention
Ch. 4, Brownlie. Cognitive development in infants. *Qualitative interviews*	✓	✓				
Ch. 5, Albertson et al. Child-bearing women in prison. *Mixed methods: Online and face to face consultation, interviews*	✓	✓			✓	
Ch. 7, Hirst. Positive sexuality and sexual health in education. *Qualitative methods*		✓				✓
Ch. 8, Formby. Wellbeing of young people who identify as lesbian, gay, bisexual or transgender. *Qualitative interviews and focus groups*		✓			✓	✓
Ch. 10, Reece and Clack. Young mums and breastfeeding. *Qualitative interviews and focus groups*	✓	✓			✓	

Ch. 11, Poll. Hepatitis C access and diagnosis. *Qualitative interviews*	✓			✓	
Ch. 13, Allmark. Welfare rights and benefits. *Realist literature review*	✓	✓		✓	
Ch. 14, Grant. Women in work and employment. *Mixed methods: survey and interviews*	✓		✓		✓
Ch. 16, Pollard. Collaborative working with the voluntary sector in chronic mental health. *Qualitative case study and interview*	✓			✓	
Ch. 17, Tod. Keeping warm in later life. *Qualitative interviews and room temperature measurements*	✓			✓	

means, seek to give expression to the lives of people who are experiencing, or are at risk of, health inequalities, or being denied social justice, power and control. Whilst the methods may not match those valued most highly in hierarchies of medical based evidence, we believe that they all contribute to the call for evidence within the Leeds Declaration. In doing so, they focus on the upstream health issues and wider health determinants, recognise lay people as experts, value plurality of methods and qualitative insight and recognise the inadequacy of experimental models (Hunter 1994).

Conclusion

This chapter has summarised the extent of the health divide in the UK that has been documented since the Black Report publication in 1980. Key headlines and priorities from public health policy and debate have been considered alongside a reflection on the contribution of the Leeds Declaration on research for public health. The next chapter considers the contribution of the work of the Marmot Review Team (2010) in providing a direction of travel for future public health policy, practice and research in addressing health inequalities.

References

Abercrombie, N., Hill, S. and Turner, B. S. (1994) *The Penguin Dictionary of Sociology*. London: Penguin Books.

Acheson, D. (1998) *The Acheson Report: Independent Inquiry into Inequalities in Health*. Online at: http://www.york.ac.uk/yhpho/documents/hea/Website/AchesonReport.pdf Accessed September 2013.

Allmark, P. and Tod, A. M. (2006) How should public health professionals engage with lay epidemiology? *Journal of Medical Ethics* 32: 460–463.

Beauchamp, D. E. (1976) Public health as social justice. *Inquiry* 13, 1 (March): 3–14.

Benzeval, M., Judge, K. and Whitehead, M. (1995) *Tackling Inequalities in Health: An Agenda for Action*. London: King's Fund.

Black, D. (1982) *Inequalities in Health: The Black Report*. London: Penguin Books.

Blaxter, M. (2004) *Health*. Oxford: Polity Press.

Busfield, J. (2000) Introduction: Rethinking the sociology of mental health. *Sociology of Health and Illness* 22, 5: 543–558.

Crowley, P. and Hunter, D. J. (2005) Putting the public back into public health. *Journal of Epidemiology and Community Health* 59: 265–267, doi:10.1136/jech.2003.019513.

Dahlgren, G. and Whitehead, M. (1991a) *Policies and Strategies to Promote Social Equity in Health*. Stockholm, Sweden: Institute for Futures Studies.

Dahlgren, G. and Whitehead, M. (1991b) What can be done about inequalities in health? *Lancet* 338, 8774: 1059–1063.

Dahlgren, G. and Whitehead, M. (2007) *European Strategies for Tackling Social Inequities in Health: Levelling Up*, Part 2. Copenhagen: WHO Regional Office for Europe.

Day, R. and Hitchings, R. (2011) 'Only old ladies would do that': age stigma and older people's strategies for dealing with winter cold. *Health Place* 17, 4: 885–894.

Department of Health (1992) *The Health of the Nation: A Strategy for Health in England*. London: HMSO.

Department of Health (1999) *Saving Lives: Our Healthier Nation*. Online at: http://www.archive. official-documents.co.uk/document/cm43/4386/4386.htm Accessed September 2012.

Department of Health (2004) *Choosing Health: Making Healthy Choices Easier.* Online at: http://webarchive.nationalarchives.gov.uk/+/dh.gov.uk/en/publicationsandstatistics/publications/publicationspolicyandguidance/dh_4094550 Accessed September 2013.

Department of Health (2009) *Tackling Health Inequalities: 2006–08 Policy and Data Update for the 2010 National Target.* Online at: http://webarchive.nationalarchives.gov.uk/+/www.dh.gov.uk/en/Publichealth/Healthinequalities/index.htm Accessed September 2013.

Department of Health (2011) *No Health Without Mental Health: A Cross-Government Mental Health Outcomes Strategy for People of All Age.* Online at: https://www.gov.uk/government/uploads/system/uploads/attachment_data/file/213761/dh_124058.pdf Accessed September 2013.

DHSS (1980) *The Black Report: Inequalities in Health: Report of a Research Working Group.* Online at: http://www.sochealth.co.uk/public-health-and-wellbeing/poverty-and-inequality/the-black-report-1980/ Accessed September 2013.

Dorling, D. (2010) Mind the gap: New Labour's legacy on child poverty. *Poverty, Journal of the Child Poverty Action Group* 136, 11–13.

Dorling, D. (2011) *Injustice: Why Social Inequalities Persist.* Bristol: Policy Press.

Doyal, L. (1995) *What Makes Women Sick: Gender and the Political Economy of Health.* London: Macmillan.

Faculty of Public Health (2010) *What is Public Health?* Online at: http://www.fph.org.uk/what_is_public_health Accessed September 2012, doi:10.1377/hlthaff.25.4.1053.

Ferrie, J. E. (ed.) (2004) *Work, Stress and Health: The Whitehall II Study.* London: International Centre for Health and Society/Department of Epidemiology and Public Health, University College; CCSU/Cabinet Office.

Gostin, L. O. and Powers, M. (2006) What does social justice require for the public's health? Public health ethics and policy imperatives. *Health Affairs* 25, 4: 1053–1060.

Graham, H. (2007) *Unequal Lives: Health and Socio-economic Inequalities.* Maidenhead, Berks: Open University Press.

Hitchings, R. and Day, R. (2011) How older people relate to the private winter warmth practices of their peers and why should we be interested. *Environment and Planning* A 43, 10: 2452–2467.

Hunter, D. (1994) Editorial – Commentary on the Leeds Declaration. *Journal of Public Health Medicine* 16, 3: 253–255.

Jones, L. (2012) Public health in context. In L. Jones and J. Douglas, *Public Health: Building Innovative Practice.* Milton Keynes: Sage.

Larsen, K. and Gilliland, J. (2008) Mapping the evolution of 'food deserts' in a Canadian city: supermarket accessibility in London, Ontario, 1961–2005. *International Journal of Health Geographics* 7: 16. doi:10.1186/1476-072X-7-16.

Long, A. F. (1993) *Understanding Health and Disease: Towards a Knowledge Base for Public Health Action.* Report of Workshop. Leeds: Nuffield Institute for Health.

Long, A. F. (1997) The Leeds Declaration: three years on – a symbol or a catalyst for change? *Critical Public Health* 7, 1–2: 73–81. Online at: http://dx.doi.org/10.1080/09581599708409080 Accessed September 2013.

Lorenc, T., Petticrew, M., Welch, V. and Tugwell, P. (2012) What types of interventions generate inequalities? Evidence from systematic reviews. *Journal of Epidemiology and Community Health.* doi:10.1136/jech-2012-201257.

Macintyre, S. (1997) The Black Report and beyond: what are the issues? *Social Science and Medicine* 44, 6: 723–745.

McKinlay, J. B. (1975) A case for refocusing upstream. The political economy of sickness. In A. J. Enelow and J. B. Henderson (eds), *Applying Behavioral Science to Cardiovascular Risk.* Washington, DC: American Heart Association.

McKinlay, J. B. and Marceau, L. D. (2000) To boldly go . . . *American Journal of Public Health* 90, 1. http://www.ncbi.nlm.nih.gov/pmc/articles/PMC1446117/pdf/10630133.pdf

Marmot Review Team (2010) *Fair Society: Healthy Lives.* Online at: http://www.instituteofhealthequity. org/projects/fair-society-healthy-lives-the-marmot-review/fair-society-healthy-lives-full-report Accessed September 2013.

Navarro, V. (2008) Neoliberalism and its consequences: the world health situation since Alma Alta. *Global Social Policy* 8, 2: 152–155.

Nazroo, J. Y. (1997) *The Health of Britain's Ethnic Minorities: Findings from a National Survey.* London: Policy Studies Institute.

Nuffield Council on Bioethics (2007) *Public Health: Ethical Issues* (2007) Online at: http://www. nuffieldbioethics.org/sites/default/files/Public%20health%20-%20ethical%20issues.pdf Accessed September 2013.

Phillipson, C. (2007) The 'elected' and the 'excluded': sociological perspectives on the experience of place and community in old age. *Ageing and Society* 27: 321–342. doi:10.1017/S0144686X06005629.

Popay, J., Thomas, C., Williams, G., Bennett, S., Gatrell, A. and Bostock, L. (2003a) A proper place to live: health inequalities, agency and the normative dimensions of space. *Social Science and Medicine* 57: 55–69.

Popay, J., Bennett, S., Thomas, C., Williams, G., Gatrell, A., and Bostock, L. (2003b) Beyond 'beer, fags, egg and chips'? Exploring lay understandings of social inequalities in health. *Sociology of Health and Illness* 25: 1–25.

Resnick, D. (2007) Responsibility for health: personal, social and environmental. *Journal of Medical Ethics* 33: 444–445.

Rose, G. (1985) Sick individuals and sick populations. *International Journal of Epidemiology* 14: 32–38.

Rose, G. (1992) *The Strategy of Preventive Medicine.* Oxford: Oxford University Press.

Scambler, G. (1997) Deviance, sick role and stigma. In G. Scambler (ed.) *Sociology as Applied to Medicine* (5th ed.). London: Saunders.

Scambler, G. (2008) *Sociology as Applied to Medicine* (6th ed.). Edinburgh: Saunders Elsevier.

Townsend, P., Davidson, N. and Whitehead, M. (1990) *Inequalities in Health: The Black Report and the Health Divide.* London: Penguin.

Wanless, D. (2002) *Securing Our Future Health: Taking a Long-Term View.* Final report. London: HM Treasury.

Wanless, D. (2004) *Securing Good Health for the Whole Population.* Final report. London: HM Treasury.

Whitehead, M. (1987) *The Health Divide: Inequalities in Health.* London: Health Education Council.

Wiley, L., Berman, M. and Blanke, D. (2013) Who's your nanny? Choice, paternalism and public health in the age of personal responsibility. *Journal of Law, Medicine and Ethics* 41 (s1), 88–91.

Wilkinson, R. and Pickett, K. (2009) *The Spirit Level.* London: Penguin.

World Health Organisation (2011) *Global Health Observatory, Life Expectancy.* Online at: http:// www.who.int/gho/mortality_burden_disease/life_tables/en/ Accessed September 2013.

2

FAIRER SOCIETY, HEALTHIER LIVES

Chris Bentley

Introduction

This chapter reflects on the Marmot Review, *Fair Society, Healthy Lives* (Marmot Review 2010), and considers its impact and role in current public health policy and practice. In this way it provides a contextual background for the content of the book's ensuing chapters. Following a summary of the development of the Review and its contribution, a critique will be provided that raises crucial questions regarding the constraints of the approach taken by Marmot and his team.

The Marmot Review: Fair Society, Healthy Lives

Sir Michael Marmot chaired the WHO Commission on the Social Determinants of Health. The final report was entitled (Commission on the Social Determinants of Health 2008) *Closing the Gap in a Generation*. This important report concluded that 'Social injustice is killing on a grand scale' (p. 34). It went on to say that health and health equity may not be the aim of all social policies but they will be a fundamental result. It distilled out three (somewhat compounded) important principles of action:

1. Improve the conditions of daily life – in which people are born, grow, live, work and age
2. Tackle the inequitable distribution of power, money and resources . . . globally, nationally and locally
3. Measure the problem, evaluate action, expand the knowledge base . . . training and awareness of the social awareness of health

As a result of positive response to the Commission Report, Sir Michael was asked by the British Government to build on it and elaborate a Strategic Review of Health Inequalities in England post-2010. The timing of this Review was tricky, coming as it did towards the end of an electoral cycle. Indeed the Report, *Fair Society, Healthy Lives* (Marmot Review 2010) was published just three months before elections led to a significant change to the political parties in government in the UK. The situation almost inevitably, and probably sensibly, favoured recommendations which were more politically neutral, as the government being asked to adopt them had very different driving principles than the one that commissioned the Review. Perhaps in consequence there was less emphasis, for example, on addressing 'inequitable distribution of power, money and resources' (Commission on the Social Determinants of Health 2008) than there otherwise might have been.

The Marmot Review, as it became known, was a grand enterprise, engaging, as it did, wide representation on its working groups from academic and service institutions and across the social sectors. The working papers drew on an extensive and varied evidence and experiential base, much of which is available as an electronic archive (Institute of Health Equity 2010). The final recommendations were placed within the conceptual framework, included as Figure 2.1.

The six main policy objectives are presented, and have been perceived, as a strong core of the recommendations. The basis of each is a robust evidence base, largely highly statistically significant quantitative data, translated into accessible, persuasive intelligence. Each of the six stands alone as a set of recommendations, but they are also linked together as a cycle of potential interventions along the 'Life Course'. The first in the sequence, 'Giving every child the best start in life', is stated as the highest priority recommendation. This should start before birth and be followed through the life of the child if the close links between early disadvantage and poor outcomes throughout life are to be broken. However, evidence is presented to show that there is much that can be done for people who have already reached school, working age and beyond. For strategies looking to intervene across the life course, the whole impact will be greater than the sum of the parts.

It is clear that this intelligence has penetrated quite widely across public health. Reference to the 'Marmot 6' is to be found in many Joint Health and Wellbeing Strategies across England.

The Marmot Review: a critique

However, as with many such reviews, 'the devil is in the delivery'. While the principles outlined are seductive, it is a major challenge to convert them into society-changing action. In many cases, the most that is achieved by many authorities and partnerships may be small project-based gestures in the direction of reduced health inequalities.

The Marmot Team dedicated Chapter 5 of their 2010 Report to 'Making it happen'. Within this, they establish two policy goals:

- Create an enabling society that maximises individual and community potential
- Ensure social justice, health and sustainability are at the heart of policies

Both goals have their place at national and local level, and at both levels, attention needs

Aim:

To reduce health inequalities and improve health and wellbeing for all

Policy goals:

1. Create an enabling society that maximises individual and community potential.
2. Ensure social justice, health and sustainability are at the heart of policies.

Policy objectives:

1. Give every child the best start in life
2. Enable all children, young people and adults, to maximise their capabilities and control their lives
3. Create fair employment and decent work for all
4. Ensure a healthy standard of living for all
5. Create and develop healthy and environmentally sustainable places and communities
6. Strengthen the role and impact of ill-health prevention

Policy mechanisms:

1. Equality and health equity in all policies
2. Effective evidence-based delivery systems

FIGURE 2.1 Conceptual framework of *Fair Society, Healthy Lives*.

to focus on how to deliver percentage change in populations, avoiding patchiness and variability. The Marmot chapter is arguably too vague in some ways, and too specific in others. It is too vague in that it does not provide principles for driving population level change. It is too specific in that most of its recommendations on delivery are addressed to structures and processes that were present at the time (e.g. Primary Care Trusts; Local Strategic Partnerships; Comprehensive Area Assessments). These were confined to history shortly after the Report was produced, as the new UK Government instituted radical programmes of reform and restructuring.

There is one fundamental principle related to delivery in the Marmot Report that is worth interrogation. It relates to Professor Marmot's concept of 'proportionate universalism' (Marmot Review 2010: 16), first established in another of his major programmes of work (Whitehall II Study 2004). This relates income deprivation score by neighbourhood to life expectancy and disability-free life expectancy (Marmot Review 2010: 11). There is a gradient across the full spectrum of deprivation. If the gradient of inequality in life expectancy is to be substantially reduced, action will be required across the whole spectrum. This is no doubt true. However, it is, arguably, the fact that the scale and intensity of action needs to be proportionate to the level of disadvantage that is potentially problematic. Those in the most deprived deciles (10 per cent), where the gradient is the steepest, tend to live in circumstances where multiple disadvantages compound together, making action on particular risks significantly harder to address. In these families and individuals, *disproportionate* inputs will be needed to make the same gains as for people in other parts of the 'gradient'. Some people need to 'climb a cliff face' before they get onto the gradient.

Whether the starting point is a biomedical or a social model of health (see Chapter 1), when it comes to attempting to deliver change, many of the principles will be similar. Issues of social justice can be pursued at an individual level, and many practitioners at the 'frontline', working at street level with individuals, families or communities will be doing just that. However, the ambition for policy and strategy is to effect changes that will be measurable or noticeable, at population level. For the Review Team, the highest priority is 'to give *every* child the best start in life' (Marmot Review 2010: 20), not just the favoured ones and others that some special projects and initiatives might reach. Translating such ideals into practice in the real world will require interventions with the power to bring about 'sea change' in circumstances and outcomes. What are the characteristics of such interventions and to what extent can policy proposals be translated into delivery systems capable of producing percentage change at population level?

Achieving health improvement for populations

This challenge was exactly the one facing the 20 per cent most deprived local authority areas with the poorest health in England, designated the 'Spearhead Areas' (Department of Health 2004). The national strategy was that these 70 named areas were, together, to be supported to reduce the mortality gap between them as a group and the national average, by 10 per cent by 2010. This did indeed require 'sea changes', and would not be achieved by any number of uncoordinated small projects, whatever their merits. As part of the strategic delivery plan, the Department of Health set up a Health Inequalities National Support Team (HINST). This Team developed and refined a number of models which would help them to appraise strategies, structures and processes, and where necessary modify them so as to obtain best possible population level outcomes from a given set of interventions. The work of HINST is now considered to explore how action to address inequalities can be scaled up to have a population effect.

The population intervention triangle

The first of these models pulled together the most significant macro mechanisms for intervention in a coherent way, allowing appraisal at the level of, for example, a local authority area. This is illustrated in Figure 2.2.

The main components of the model are the following:

Population level interventions. These are macro level actions which help make 'healthy choices easier choices' for individuals. They include legislation, regulation, taxation, licensing and public media campaigns. They also include healthy public policy. This

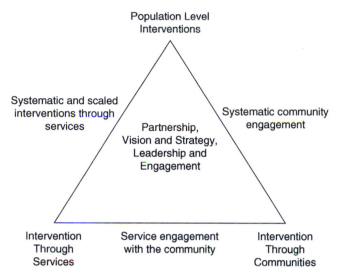

FIGURE 2.2 Producing percentage change at population level (Bentley 2011).

crosses the sectors, e.g. education; welfare benefits; housing; transport and crime and community safety, and can be driven by mechanisms such as Health Impact and Equity Impact Assessments (Scott-Samuel 2001). This level of intervention, although usually intended to encompass all relevant parts of the population, cannot be assumed to do so. To achieve equal coverage and equitable impact, it will be necessary to evaluate penetration of effect, particularly to target vulnerable groups, and to follow up appropriately with selective education, advice, support and, where necessary, enforcement (for examples see Chapters 13 and 17).

Interventions through services. Many evidence-based interventions work well at the level of the individual, when delivered appropriately and effectively. The medication called a statin, for example, when taken regularly by someone found to have raised cholesterol in their blood (associated with heart disease), can reduce their chance of a heart attack or a stroke by 30–40 per cent (Wright 1994). In theory, if there were enough of these individual successes, the cumulative impact could add up to a percentage change in mortality at population level. However, HINST experience showed that in many communities, the system and scale in services necessary to build up that cumulative impact were often missing. This problem was made worse in that it was, commonly, the most disadvantaged, often most at risk, that were missing out. This lack of system and scale in delivery can often be seen across the range of services, for example affordable warmth initiatives and benefits advice, as subsequent chapters will illustrate.

Interventions through communities. Individuals and families are much influenced by the communities they are part of. Communal knowledge and understanding helps form individual awareness of what can help or harm wellbeing and health, as well as expectations of life in general, and of services in particular. Peer support and pressure will influence behaviours people exhibit, beliefs and practices that are acceptable, and actions to take. The term 'community' (literally the 'gift of being together') can cover a range of groupings, for example community of place (neighbourhood), community of interest (religious and cultural groups; clubs and societies) and communities of practice (schools; workplaces; professional groups). Obviously the categories have significant overlaps. Groupings as diverse as farming communities and gangs may be brought together on issues related to place, interest or practice. The development of the internet has widened the nature of connectivity in a virtual world, so that social connections and influences can be established without the members of such communities ever needing to meet.

If those seeking to influence the social determinants of health could engage with, and influence, such communities, their strengths could be harnessed to influence knowledge, behaviours and outcomes of those who belong. There are arguably three main categories of community engagement, each of which may have their place in population-based strategies.

- *Consultation:* engaging communities to obtain their input, perspectives and ideas on vision, strategy and plans. Discussions should avoid being tokenistic, and attempt to draw in otherwise 'seldom seen, seldom heard' elements of the community. Good examples have involved the development of peer researchers from within the community to draw out community intelligence (Turning Point 2013). Where possible the dialogue should be ongoing, with the capability of influencing the *delivery* of planned programmes.
- *Partnership:* this involves a sharing of power over the outcome of the intervention. Figuratively, representatives of all those engaging in a process should be equitably represented and, in principle or in reality, have equal 'voting rights'. Ownership of the process and the outcomes of engagement should be shared.
- *Empowerment:* this (least common) form of engagement involves a transfer of significant power and/or resources from external agencies to the community itself. It may involve a form of commissioning whereby a desired outcome is negotiated and agreed, but what is planned, and how it should be done, is left mostly to local discretion. This form of engagement is usually an expression of mature relationships, and requires a good degree of confidence in the leadership, capability and organisational ability of the community itself (Turning Point 2013).

Whichever its style, HINST found community engagement, even within a given local authority, to be patchy and variable. Policy initiatives prioritising, encouraging and supporting it had been episodic at national and regional levels. Significant resourcing had appeared in waves, being favoured in times of plenty, but among the first type of initiative to go in times of austerity and public sector cuts.

On a local basis, expression of the use of budgets for community development would frequently take the form of a contest, whereby there would be an invitation to submit bids against a tender. It was usual that communities that were successful would be those that already had good leadership, organisation, social cohesion and ideas, hence they could submit attractive bids. Depressed communities with few attributes and assets, often the most needy, would once again miss out, and be left behind.

Addressing inequalities in outcomes at population level requires such communities to be targeted for disproportionate support. They will need preparatory work before they can even get onto the field of play. They may need support with 1, asset mapping; 2, identification and development of leadership candidates; 3, initiatives to develop social capital and cohesion; and 4, supported community-based research to help identify and boost local aspiration and raise levels of expectation. These approaches can work very effectively, for example in Sheffield, where the Health Action Zone funded such preparation as a first phase in a number of target neighbourhoods, at the same time as supporting some of the worthy but 'usual suspects' to get immediately up and running. By phases two and three communities in preparation were 'job ready', and able to take on programmes of their own devising. Unfortunately, in terms of the Marmot thesis, it is indisputable that at community level there needs to be some 'disproportionate' input before there can be 'universalism'.

Service engagement with communities. HINST experience again (Smithies 2010) showed that many 'frontline' services, although doing good work for those that crossed their thresholds, often functioned in splendid isolation from the community in which they were based. Within primary care, there were examples of general practitioners/physicians (GPs) putting in a full day of good quality work ministering to those coming through their waiting rooms. They may have been providing good quality personal care, but on many occasions were heard to say they were 'too busy' to go looking for extra work. Others, however, were concerned to find and draw in the 'missing', who may have been the neediest, but lacking the knowledge, self-esteem, expectations and even skills to seek appropriate, timely help. These proactive practitioners were able to organise their general practice resources accordingly, and, in particular, connect with contacts and infrastructures in the community itself, as well as other public health 'partner' services, such as social care, housing, benefits agencies and the police.

Critical in developing the linkages between services and communities of all sorts, is the 'Third Sector'. This is mainly an aggregation of voluntary, community and faith organisations in this context; they often have grown out of, or represent, communities and their particular needs. They will also work with, and often provide components of, services. In support of individual health and wellbeing they can be critical, often providing more accessible and approachable, tailored and user friendly services than (what may be seen as) the more daunting, bureaucratic and inflexible public sector. From a population health and wellbeing perspective, however, there can be weaknesses. In any given area, an aggregation of agencies may not function as a sector, being instead fragmented, variable and inconsistent. In terms of strategic intent to make a percentage difference at population level, it is often difficult to harness its heterogeneity, and so to bring interventions to bear as required with system and scale.

This can be done, however, and there are many examples where it has been achieved with success. Some of the principles have been pulled together to lay out the framework for a systematic process (Grahame 2010).

The population intervention triangle described above outlines the various mechanisms capable of delivering percentage change at population level. It will be critical for those looking to deliver the recommendations of the Marmot Review at local level to give full consideration to the principles involved if they are to produce more than low-level change. Preferably, they will be used in combination to produce multi-hit strategies generating holistic societal change.

The decay model of uptake across delivery pathways

The Marmot Review recommends a wide range of interventions and support to be delivered 'across the social gradient'. In order to achieve this it is important to understand the reasons why this has not been achieved substantially in the past.

An important model of the effective uptake of evidence-based interventions is given as Figure 2.3(a) (Harrison et al. 2006). This has shown that there is a tendency for only a small percentage of people who could possibly benefit to actually achieve the desirable results of the treatment or therapy. This is demonstrated in relation to a variety of long-term conditions that are ongoing challenges for public health and demonstrates a consistent number of stages of 'decay' in the potential benefit being achieved.

Assuming that such a pathway is likely to exist in relation to a whole range of potential inputs, it will then be important to systematically try to address the various stages of 'programme decay', so as to maximise the impact that the evidence-based interventions can have on as many as possible with a given health and social care need. Figure 2.3(b), therefore identifies four such stages, A–D, which can be the focus for population-based programmes to deliver interventions to those vulnerable in any given population

A. *Knowledge and understanding*: This component of strategy relates to knowledge and understanding of a given problem, which will influence action taken. There are a number of factors that will determine how this understanding is distributed across a community (Athey et al. 2011; Tod et al. 2001), including:

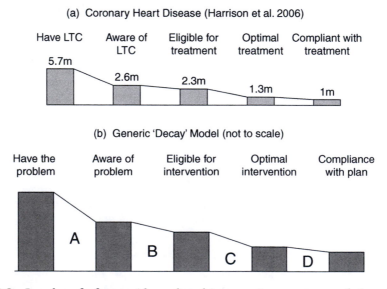

(a) Coronary Heart Disease (Harrison et al. 2006)

Have LTC   Aware of   Eligible for   Optimal   Compliant with
           LTC   treatment   treatment   treatment

5.7m

2.6m   2.3m   1.3m   1m

(b) Generic 'Decay' Model (not to scale)

Have the   Aware of   Eligible for   Optimal   Compliance
problem   problem   intervention   intervention   with plan

A   B   C   D

FIGURE 2.3 Lost benefit from evidence-based interventions across populations (Harrison et al. 2006).

- Community knowledge, understanding, beliefs and expectation: about condition, about services, about life; and stigma;
- Personal beliefs and skills: demotivation; low expectations; low self-confidence; poor literacy; low IQ, etc.

B. *Presentation and case-finding*: By what mechanisms do cases of need come to the attention of services? These will include direct self-referral; referral from other services; outreach; screening and other case-finding approaches. Service factors having an impact (Athey et al. 2011) include:

- Geographical, e.g. distance from service outlet, clinic/practice; complex journey; lack of money for fare;
- User unfriendly service access: frosty, bureaucratic reception; cultural/interpreter problems; perceived discrimination; expectation of judgement; appointment systems; access delays; opening hours; cost barriers.

C. *Service effectiveness and quality*: Once engaged with the service, how effectively are the right interventions matched to the right problems, and implemented in the right way? This will depend on a range of factors (Leaman 2010), including:

- Inefficient service – are management systems in place to best support the service user and practitioner?
- Ineffective practitioner – are they accredited and well trained, with systems of audit, governance, support? and appraisal in place to keep them up to date, well informed, skilled and safe?
- Unresponsive service – not committed to outcome. Are services pro-active, driving for best outcomes for the user and the service, rather than passive, reacting only to user demand?

D. *Support for self-management*: Most interventions depend to a large extent on the inputs of users themselves, with only a small percentage of intervention time spent with a supportive practitioner. This is true for management of a medical condition, e.g. diabetes; behaviour change, e.g. weight loss; moderated drinking/abstinence or social determinants, e.g. education/money management/affordable warmth.
Key elements include:

- The user should be part of any decision making about their 'care' plan.
- One-size-fits-all education/self-management support will not accommodate the variety of skills, preferences and learning styles.
- Use of peer and community support from those with similar issues.

Conclusion

The Marmot Report is an important basis for future action to address social injustice and the social determinants of health. It lays out a strong, largely epidemiological, evidence base, well analysed and clearly presented, which identifies many of the fundamental problems, and points the way to the kind of actions that will need to be taken to address them.

However, as mentioned above, 'the devil will be in delivery'. Each of the interventions identified by the Marmot Team will be only one of the active ingredients of programmes delivered in complex and varied environments. Understanding of the complexity will require substantial other forms of local inquiry to augment the epidemiology. Multiple methods and multiple perspectives are needed to understand health problems and to result in action. Particular emphasis will need to be placed on capture and use of lay knowledge (Leeds Declaration).

This chapter has described key models which provide systematic frameworks to support how interventions in complex environments can be planned so as to give a strong basis for optimal measurable change at population level. Examples of research and insight work addressing components of these strategic issues are given in subsequent chapters of this book. They will seek to illustrate how strong qualitative research can help drive progress towards Fair society, Healthy lives.

References

Athey, V. L., Suckling, R., Tod, A. M., Walters, S. J. and Rogers, T. K. (2011) Early diagnosis of lung cancer: evaluation of a community-based social marketing intervention. *Thorax* 67: 412–417. doi:10.1136/thoraxjnl-2011-200714.

Bentley, C. (2011) *A Generic Diagnostic Framework for Addressing Inequalities in Outcome at Population Level from Evidence-based Interventions*. London: Health Inequalities National Support Team, Department of Health.

Commission on the Social Determinants of Health (2008) *Closing the Gap in a Generation*. Geneva: WHO, World Health Organisation.

Department of Health (2004, November 19) Reid announces 'Spearhead' PCTs to tackle health inequalities. News release. London: Department of Health.

Grahame, N. (2010) *How to Develop the Third (Voluntary, Community and Faith) Sector as a Strategic Partner*. London: Health Inequalities National Support Team, Department of Health.

Harrison, W., Marshal, T., Singh, D. and Tennant, R. (2006) *The Effectiveness of Healthcare Systems in the UK-Scoping Study*. Birmingham: Department of Public Health and Epidemiology and HEMC, University of Birmingham.

Institute of Health Equity (2010, February) *Marmot Review Task Group Reports*. Online at: http://www.instituteofhealthequity.org/projects/marmot-review-task-groups Accessed 19 May 2013.

Leaman, J. (2010) *Raising the Bar in Primary Care*. London: Health Inequalities National Support Team, Department of Health.

Marmot Review (2010) *Fair Society, Healthy Lives*. London: The Marmot Review.

Scott-Samuel, A. B. (2001) *The Merseyside Guidelines for Health Impact Assessment* (2nd ed.). Liverpool: International health IMPACT Assessment Consortium.

Smithies, J. (2010) *Customer Access Strategies: Developing Targeted Services to Increase Accessibility*. London: Health Inequalities National Support Team, Department of Health.

Tod, A. M., Read, C., Lacey, A. and Abbott, J. (2001) Overcoming barriers to uptake of services for coronary heart disease: a qualitative study. *British Medical Journal* 323: 214–217.

Turning Point (2013) *Explaining Connected Care: Doing Things Differently*. London: Turning Point.

Whitehall II Study (2004) *Work, Stress and Health: The Whitehall II Study*. London: Council for the Civil Service Unions/Cabinet Office.

Wright, A. R. (1994) The Scandinavian Simvastatin Study (4S). *Lancet* 344, 8939: 1765–1768.

3

PRE-BIRTH AND EARLY YEARS (UP TO AGE FIVE)

Chris Bentley

Introduction

The findings and recommendations of the Marmot Review are structured on the framework of the 'Life Course'. Fundamental to this is that the consequences of social, psychological, economic and environmental influences accumulate through life's phases to have a combined impact. The evidence from the Review, however, is that it can be the impact of what happens in the Early Years that 'casts the longest shadow'. The effects can either be:

- *Protective* – increasing esteem; life skills; resilience and behaviours
- *Hazardous* – destroying self-regard; undermining social skills and ability to learn; creating the conditions for mental and physical ill health. (Marmot Review 2010: 40)

One of the most striking findings of the whole Review relates to cognitive development. In summary 'Children of educated or wealthy parents can score poorly in early tests but still catch up, whereas children of worse-off parents are unlikely to do so' (Marmot Review 2010: 61–62). A range of empirical studies are pointed to which provide evidence that cognitive ability is a powerful determinant of earnings, propensity to get involved in crime *(or not)*, and success *(or otherwise)* in many aspects of social and economic life as well as health, across the social gradient (Marmot Review 2010: 61–62).

Shifting the focus from education to relationship to support vulnerable infants and their parents

Our first chapter highlighting a specific study based on research (Chapter 4) makes the case that probably as important as cognitive development in the early years, and strongly interacting with it, are components of emotional and social development. Marmot alludes to this as 'also important', being 'development of non-cognitive skills such as application, self-regulation and empathy', without describing any strong evidence in support.

In Chapter 4 Brownlie builds on the importance of these as critical executive functioning skills which will have a profound lifelong impact on neurological, emotional, social, physical, communication and behavioural development.

With better understanding of the place of executive skills as part of the foundations of development comes the need to explore how it might be possible to support their better development in vulnerable infants, if they are to break out of the cycles of deprivation. The chapter makes clear that there is a good basis of scientific understanding and some good examples of systems for its practical application, but dissemination and use of this valuable knowledge and its associated skills is patchy and variable.

In considering how it might be possible to achieve a population level change in the distribution of support for the development of executive functioning in infants, it is necessary to consider the 'population intervention triangle' described in Chapter 2 of this book. Brownlie brings some focus to bear on two apices of that triangle.

The first is population level intervention through policy, at the top of the triangle, aiming to achieve a 'systemic revolution' to meet the needs of infants (and their parents/carers). The key policy initiative providing the basis for this has been to extend the duty of local authorities to secure early years provision free of charge for two-year-olds living in low income households (from September 2013 in England). While this is potentially an important step in supporting early years development at population level, the case is made here that other development needs of vulnerable children need to be at the core of the initiative, not just 'enriched education'. It is suggested that if the full benefit of this worthy initiative is to be attained, it will be necessary to gain ownership across policy departments at national and local levels of government and organisation. It will also be necessary to bring together knowledge base and practice across a number of current cultural silos, e.g. education and infant mental health.

Action to achieve such a goal could well be driven from another apex of the population intervention triangle: systematic and scaled-up changes in service delivery. An important method to achieve this is through application of consistent, quality assured and appropriate training. The piece of research described here by Brownlie would help to support application of just such a training intervention. The training itself is short and sharp. In what could be a very theoretically complex area, the focus is described on two core skills, attunement and regulation, brought together in one model of good practice, the Solihull Approach. The study explores whether these components provide childminders in training with effective knowledge, skills and some tools to augment their practice. If it does so, the training provides potential to improve outcomes for vulnerable children, for their parents, and also for the practitioners themselves.

Strong qualitative research on the impact of such an initiative should help make the case to expand its use from a small project to a programme aiming for application with system, scale and sustainability.

Addressing health inequalities for mothers and babies in prison: findings from a consultation exercise

In Chapter 5 of this book, Albertson focuses on a small but extremely vulnerable group of mothers and their children. The women themselves are a strongly biased sample of those with socially deprived backgrounds, many suffering the results of mental illness, addiction and abuse. While there may be concerns therefore about the quality of the 'early start' available to the children in the ante-natal, perinatal and infancy periods, there may also be opportunities if best use can be made of mothers in prison being a 'captive audience'.

The piece of research described identifies high levels of experience, expertise and enthusiasm among both prison and health sector staff to support both mothers and their babies during this 'crucial life stage'. However, this is patchy and a very mixed picture emerges. The research here helps to identify how a more systematic population based approach could potentially change this substantially.

In terms of the population intervention triangle, attention should be focused at the centre, identifying possibilities to improve leadership, partnership and vision and strategy.

Leadership: although there are only relatively few Mother and Baby Units (MBUs) in English prisons, and practitioners within these do communicate with each other, there has been little formalised joint working across units to enable shared learning about good practice and models of care. There is an opportunity in England to put this right, as the responsibility for specialty commissioning of offender/prison health has been centralised under NHS England. This body will 'provide the frameworks to ensure consistency of commissioning'. It 'will draw on nationwide insight and intelligence and reflect innovation, clinical knowledge and expertise . . .' (NHS Commissioning Board 2013: 20–21).

Partnership: despite the good intentions of some practitioners, the study identifies a range of factors which militate against success, including cultures of working and lack of understanding of organisational constraints between agencies such as health and prison services, and between prison and community services. Again this may be facilitated by the Local Area Teams of NHS England as part of their remit to help manage local relationships (NHS Commissioning Board 2013: 21).

Vision and strategy: this will need to be jointly developed and owned across a number of sectors if practical models of care and action plans are to be developed. Ideally these should be based on jointly agreed measures of outcome. The study identifies a range of important issues about sharing evidence, sharing data and intelligence, and communication, if joint strategy is to be a reality.

Importantly this study begins to demonstrate how eminently do-able systems and bureaucracy changes could result in improved outcomes across the life course for a very vulnerable group of individuals.

References

Marmot Review (2010) *Fair Society, Healthy Lives.* London: The Marmot Review.

NHS Commissioning Board (2013) Securing Excellence in Commissioning for Offender Health. London: NHS.

4

GIVING CHILDREN THE BEST START

Shifting the focus from education to relationship in order to support vulnerable infants and their parents

Zoe Brownlie

Introduction

Marmot states that the key priority for addressing health inequalities is to, 'Give every child the best start in life'. This chapter explores some of the key processes required to implement this objective and the essential qualities which make a difference to children's early years health and development. As Marmot recognises, action is required across agencies to address health inequalities. The question underpinning this chapter is whether key processes within the infant mental health literature can be shared in childcare settings to improve practice and children's wellbeing. Currently educational perspectives dominate in the majority of childcare settings in relation to improving children's health and wellbeing.

This chapter examines a staff training programme with child-minders who are about to receive vulnerable two-year-old children into their care. The training was designed by the author with reference to other programmes (Booth and Jenberg 2010; Crittenden 2013; Gerhardt 2004; Hughes and Baylin 2012; Solihull Primary Care Trust 2004). The purpose of the training programme is to increase the child-minder's understanding of vulnerable infants and the importance of relationship work to enable the infant's development of empathy and self-regulation. It also aims to increase the child-minder's confidence in supporting parents. The evaluation will look at the impact of the training on the child-minder's knowledge, practice and professional identity.

Underpinning theory and policy

Theory and evidence

Current evidence supports the premise that the first years of life are critical to the future life chances of an individual (Barlow et al. 2010; Shonkoff and Phillips 2000). The infant mental health literature suggests that the key protective factor for children's long-term health, wellbeing and development is the quality of the interactions that they receive. It is through their experience of relationships that infants develop a sense of self, an understanding of others and an internal working model which they bring to all aspects of their lives (Gerhardt 2004). Stresses on the caregiver/child relationship may be due to adult, child or social factors, though the child relies on the carer's ability to regulate the demands to be able to offer sensitive, appropriate care to them (Child Psychotherapy Trust 2002).

Empathy, self-regulation, attention, sociability and motivation are well-embedded patterns in a child's brain by the age of three (Zeedyck 2011). These are the foundations for the development of executive functioning within the brain. The quality of the development of the child's executive functioning skills will have a profound lifelong impact on their neurological, emotional, social, physical, communication and behavioural development and it is now argued these early experiences also impact on the immune system (Karr-Morse and Wiley 2012; Shonkoff and Garner 2011).

Clinical theorising suggests that the key processes which influence the quality of relationships are 'attunement', 'regulation' and 'structure' (predictable environments) (Perry 2002; Solihull Primary Care Trust 2004). A child who does not have good enough experiences of these processes is more likely to experience chronic stress. One result of chronic stress on the developing brain is that the brain becomes over-reliant on the limbic system. These children become hyper-vigilant in their interactions as their 'alarm system' is hardwired to activate quickly (Hughes 2012; Perry 2004). Unless these children's relationships improve they will continue to struggle to access their thinking, rational brain at times of even moderate stress as they respond in a protective but defensive way. In turn, this contributes to disruptions in future relationships and learning. The key protective factor for these children is to receive care from someone who is able to help the children regulate their arousal state and be attuned to their individual needs as this will enable them to develop the required executive functioning skills. This becomes more challenging, the more defensive the child.

A plethora of policy documents, both nationally and internationally, have been published over the last ten years that stress the critical importance of investing in the early years so as to strengthen the foundations of children's development such as Supporting Families in the Foundation Years (Department for Education and Department of Health 2011) and the Healthy Child Programme (Department of Health 2009). The purpose is to benefit both the individual and society as a whole, as evidence demonstrates benefits at a social and economic level (Heckman 2011; The WAVE Trust and DfE 2013a, 2013b). These policies also recognise that parents require support to give children good enough care. Marmot recognises that we need to create the conditions to enable parents to develop healthy relationships in the child's critical first years and encourages staff development in this area.

However, implementation of this theoretical knowledge is inevitably shaped by the existing structures which deliver children's services and the political and economic context of the time. To fully address the needs of vulnerable infants, investment and collaboration are required across health, education and social care systems, together with child and adult services. Commissioning of services for children within England and Wales is complicated by budgets being held within separate departments. Kennedy (2010) notes that fundamental differences in departmental philosophy manifest themselves as tensions, as policy is translated into practice from national, to regional and local level. Kennedy quotes one senior official as reporting to him that 'You might think that the DCSF[1] and the [Department of Health] don't work for the same Government' (Kennedy 2010: 49). Marmot calls for effective local delivery systems focused on health equity in all policies in order to bring about effective change.

The dominant resource for children services is education. However, traditionally education has limited evidence, theoretical knowledge and choice of interventions to address the complex social and psychological needs of individual vulnerable infants. Though classrooms across the country are significantly impacted upon by children with poor executive functioning skills (research suggests at least 15 per cent of children suffer significant chronic stress (Bayer et al. 2007; NSPCC 2011)), staff are given little understanding or capacity to deal with their needs. Moreover, the system can, at times, further alienate these children and deepen their inability to regulate themselves, feel valued or understood. There is a risk that, if children's struggles are understood as simple behavioural problems and initial behavioural approaches fail to solve the problem, the child's difficulties becomes more entrenched, leading to greater disruptions in learning throughout the child's life.

One eminent expert, James Heckman, Nobel Laureate in Economic Sciences, states:

> An important lesson to draw from the entire literature on successful early interventions is that it is the social skills and motivation of the child that are more easily altered – not IQ. These social and emotional skills affect performance in school and in the workplace. We too often have a bias toward believing that only cognitive skills are of fundamental importance to success in life.
>
> *(Heckman 2000: 7)*

The argument for a systemic revolution to meet the needs of infants is gathering pace (WAVE Trust and DfE 2013a, 2013b). Meanwhile, children's services continue to struggle to be more proactive in early intervention. It is difficult to prioritise preventative work at a time of economic restraint. Limited resources have difficulty redirecting their efforts as they struggle to ameliorate entrenched problems. The NSPCC (2011) estimates up to 20 per cent of young people are struggling with significant traumatic experiences. The system is embroiled in the need to keep 'fire fighting' without having the resources to minimise the cause of the 'fire'. For example the Department of Health's spending on Child and Adolescent Mental Health Services (CAMHS) is said to be £523 million. The social care budget is £4 billion. The spending on children and young people (up to age 25) by the criminal justice system is said to be £7 billion. The budget for education is £35.4 billion (Kennedy 2010).

The fact that children's services are commissioned via different departments, and thus budgets, reduces the incentive for one department to invest heavily in early intervention and prevention as the economic benefit to them may not be obvious, i.e. greater investment by the NHS to address issues in the early years will initially benefit education. Why would the criminal justice system offer to give up a proportion of their budget, given that they have no expertise in early years work, in order to reduce the risk for children becoming involved in anti-social behaviour and crime at a later age? As evidence gathers, one hopes that greater awareness of these issues nationally and within local authorities will drive through the diversion of funds from symptomatic to proactive investment.

Kennedy (2010) states that we need to overcome what he describes as cultural barriers within the NHS so as to better meet the needs of children and young people. He states that the problems that children and young people encounter are more often than not the product of the interaction of a variety of social forces, meaning that the response to their needs has to be equally multi-faceted (Kennedy 2010). He calls for an amalgamation of children's services so all are invested in wanting to resource early intervention at the earliest opportunity, thus reducing more ingrained problems further down the line.

The policy agenda

A key policy initiative to try and meet the needs of the most vulnerable infants has been to extend the duty of local authorities to secure free early years provision (Department for Education 2012) for two-year-olds living in low income households from September 2013. This is a popular political intervention. Not only does it address the early years agenda, it also attempts to tackle childhood poverty as it provides a means to get parents back to work. However, there is a danger that this will not address the actual needs of vulnerable infants, as they require sensitive healthy relationships from someone who cares about their individual needs. Shonkoff (2011) warns that the needs of vulnerable children are not simply met by enriched education. The government's eligibility criteria for 'vulnerable infants' is defined by family income, although, of course, many families on low incomes offer appropriate sensitive parenting. Moreover, research suggests that the incidence of children experiencing chronic stress from inappropriate parenting cuts across all socio-economic groups (Bayer et al. 2007). The author defines vulnerable infants as those who are experiencing chronic stress within their dominant relationships.

Educational systems generally rely on children having good enough executive functioning skills, in line with their developmental age, to benefit from the learning environment. Skills such as impulse control, concentration, flexibility in thinking, and managing social relationships begin to develop in the early years. However, the most at risk children may have specific delays in these skills, even at age two. It is therefore important that early years educational providers understand the critical importance of attuned relationships and how to address a child's regulation needs alongside the need to provide a predictable environment (structure) in order to develop the healthy foundations for these children's future wellbeing and learning (Perry 2002).

The research and its findings

The training

The training described in this chapter was originally developed by a local authority (Adair 2009), and is now part of the accreditation process of the child-minders being able to receive funded places for vulnerable two-year-old children (as defined by the government's eligibility criteria in 2012) coming into their care. Three days of training was delivered to 35 child-minders over two cohorts. The evaluation looks at the impact of the training on the child-minders' knowledge, practice and professional identity. It explores whether the concepts from the infant mental health literature are useful within a childcare context (see Figure 4.1). The key concepts introduced were 'attunement' and 'regulation'. It was also hoped that the training would support the child-minders' partnerships with parents through reference to the Solihull Approach (Solihull Primary Care Trust 2004) a communication model which utilises these concepts.

Data on the child-minders' experience of the training was collected from those attending the training through focused discussion and written feedback. All data have been anonymised. Thematic analysis was carried out on the data to capture each child-minder's experience of the training and understanding of the concepts introduced. The overwhelming feedback was that they found the concepts enhanced their current practice, supported their confidence in their role and gave them an extra set of tools to best support vulnerable children and their parents.

Impact on the child-minding role

The child-minders aspired to offer the children in their care a homely, caring environment where they could respond flexibly to a child's needs and offer intensive one-to-one support.

Key topics	Explanation
Attunement	Attunement is essentially about being in tune with another. Appropriate attunement enhances an infant's learning and development as they feel valued, understood, heard and validated. It helps them to organise their thinking and make sense of their needs and how to meet these needs. It develops their resourcefulness and resilience, and enables development. In order to offer appropriate attunement it is important to take time to listen and observe in order to understand the other.
Regulation	Regulation is the ability to adjust our internal state to cope with external demands. It enables us to remain within optimal levels of arousal so we can be rational, coherent and reflective in our thinking. Infants need support from their caregivers to regulate themselves, and through receiving appropriate levels of regulation they will begin to develop strategies to self-regulate.
The Solihull Approach	A model of communication which combines learning from attunement, regulation and structure as a means to provide appropriate care for infants, appropriate staff support for parents and appropriate support for staff themselves.

FIGURE 4.1 Key themes of the child-minder training.

Collectively, child-minders identified the key qualities of their role as being:

- friendly, approachable, fun, spontaneous, caring, loving, homely, understanding, kind, enthusiastic, willing to learn, organised, reliable, patient, calm, able to listen to children, diligent, flexible, able to offer 1:1; a key person, playful, give choice.

Participants identified the child's needs as being:

- routine, care, activity, love, attention, hygiene, healthy food, play, sleep, stability, choice, safety, home environment, learning, fun, equality, time.

Following the training the child-minders reported that having a greater understanding of 'attunement', 'regulation' and the needs of vulnerable children had helped them feel more confident in their role. These concepts offered a theoretical framework which supported their current practice. It was particularly helpful when they experienced challenges within their role and were less able to retain the qualities of childminding they aspired to.

> Make me more competent and confident.
>
> *(Jo)*

> Helps me become the outstanding child-minder I am always aiming to become.
>
> *(Angela)*

> Understanding children in the best way possible. Enabling me to provide good quality childcare.
>
> *(Amanda)*

Before the training started the child-minders collectively described their main challenges as being:

- Paper work, Ofsted,[2] being isolated.
- Parents: concern about parenting, different expectations regarding discipline, lack of discipline, non-payment, unrealistic demands, being late, separation issues, parent's terminal illness, use of car, safeguarding.
- Children: juggling children's needs; having happy children; challenging behaviour: not sharing, throwing toys, hitting others, squabbling, biting, scratching, aggressive behaviour; separation issues; communication delay; death in the family; low muscle tone; no English.

The data collected prior to the training suggested that when the child-minders felt challenged by difficult discussions with parents or by a child's behaviour their ideals were compromised. It would appear from the child-minders' report that they were more likely to become judgemental of the parents and feel pressured to persevere with rigid behavioural strategies with the children.

Understanding the needs of parents

The child-minders felt they could offer parents: 'A friendly approach, available day and night, not certain, gave choice and parent terminated contract, explanation, talk to parents, comfort, confidence, inform them of policy/experience.'

Before the training participants were asked to describe what 'issues' they had with parents and to state what they thought were the parents' needs at this time. It was interesting that the child-minders struggled to put themselves in the parents' shoes but, rather, referred to what they felt the parents needed to do to better support them as child-minders: 'They need to know I have bills to pay, feel safe about child-minder; for me to fulfil their demands; understand my needs; comfort and reassurance; acknowledgement of issue' (Deb).

After the training the child-minders appeared to shift towards a more empathic and considered approach regarding the needs of the parents. They reported that it was helpful to have a conceptual framework to appreciate how a parent's alarm system may be triggered when they focused on concerns about their child. They recognised that it was important for both the parents and the child-minder themselves to feel regulated, so they were able to engage in coherent, rational discussions to develop appropriate solutions. The child-minders also identified that it is important for them to offer attunement to the child and parent in order to understand each of their needs and to keep an open mind as to what the issues may be.

Post-training feedback that illustrates this new insight includes the following:

> I am pleased that I understand the importance of helping children to calm down but also helping young teenage parents who have struggles. I have had difficult conversations and this training will help me to practice skills.
>
> *(Jo)*

> This training I hope will make me effective as a practitioner to support parents to have a 'thinking head' once regulated using the skills so they can help their child.
>
> *(Amanda)*

> It will improve my confidence in dealing with difficult situations/conversations with parents.
>
> *(Sarah)*

The importance of the concepts of attunement and regulation

During the training it became obvious that the child-minders had a wealth of experience and commitment to offer a caring secure environment to the children in their care. Occasionally they came across a child's behaviour which they found to be particularly challenging. It was then their own sense of competence was challenged. The dominant paradigm in these situations is to adopt pure behaviour management strategies. However, the child-minders sensed that this was not always effective. One child-minder stated that she aimed to give the children in her care 'the best day' and therefore felt demoralised if there had been struggles with a child's challenging behaviour throughout the day.

The child-minders reported that they found the concepts of attunement and regulation complemented the behaviour management strategies already within their repertoire and helped them to have a wider choice of interventions at challenging times. The child-minders spoke of how understanding these concepts meant they felt less guilty and concerned that their actions could be perceived as condoning a child's behaviour.

> Helps make the day run smoother. Helps me deal with situations/tantrums better.
>
> *(Deb)*

> Helps me to not feel guilty about feeling I am condoning a child's behaviour even though I empathise with them.
>
> *(Kim)*

The core concepts in the training helped the child-minders to think more carefully about a child's unique complex needs and those of the parent. It gives emphasis to the need to take time to assess and observe, to meet the child's needs for regulation and also to think about their own needs. Observation and assessment are key areas of the early years foundation stage profile but there the focus is more on monitoring the child's developmental level rather than trying to understand the child's emotional world and needs:

> Makes me focus more on individual needs and planning around that. Gives me confidence to handle negative behaviours in a positive way.
>
> *(Kim)*

> My own practice – to reflect on emotions, how I deal with them in situations.
>
> *(Sarah)*

> The Solihull Approach was very helpful. Looking at regulation, behaviour and attunement.
>
> *(Amanda)*

The concept of attunement helped the child-minders understand the amount of learning which happens between people and how this process promotes development. It is important for a child to feel connected and understood by another to help them to understand their own emotional world and build their resilience. It also helps those caring for a child to adapt their demands and expectations so as to work within the child's zone of proximal development which gives the child the best opportunity for development and learning.

> I have begun to mirror my children more. It made me re-think some of the relationships with the children I have. We are quite a busy setting and it made me realise I have been not so in tune with some of the quieter children or dismissing the ones that are quite demanding. I have tried copying them in play etc. and it has made a real difference to our interactions.
>
> *(Emma)*

Regulation helped the child-minders deal with children who are dysregulating, as well as understanding the stresses the parents may be experiencing.

> Importance to wait for someone to calm down so they are able to access their thinking brain and act more rationally, rather than dash in with advice or behaviour management.
>
> *(Sarah)*

> It will make me think carefully about why the child is reacting in the way he/she does and my responses to that. Makes me want to learn more about it.
>
> *(Kath)*

> Remembering to explain emotions to young children who might not realise what they are feeling, i.e. anger, jealousy, fear.
>
> *(Gill)*

It was extremely valuable for the child-minders to understand that arousal states fluctuate and that they can help teach and support a child's ability to self-regulate. This insight encouraged the child-minders to reflect on their own needs for regulation and ensure they have enough support to cope with the demands of the role.

Application to practice

To reiterate, Marmot specifically states that the key priority to reduce health inequalities is to give every child the best start in life. Even by the age of two some children have already got off to a 'rocky start' as early experience of chronic stress impacts on their ability to cope and learn. Addressing the needs of these vulnerable children is not just about providing them with enriched learning opportunities but it is also about understanding their specific emotional and cognitive needs. Focusing on the critical importance of relationships enables children to have a healthier inner world. This will impact on their life chances. It is also important to address the needs of their parents to maximise the possibility of them receiving appropriate support to offer good enough parenting. This evaluation of a training intervention, though limited, suggests that learning from the infant mental health literature can be of value in supporting childcare workers' ability to best meet children's needs.

Childcare provision is a popular intervention for infants identified as vulnerable. It is helpful if staff within these settings understand children's complex emotional needs and draw on a range of evidence. This fits with Marmot's call for greater multi-agency working; more effective local delivery and proportionate universalism as these concepts are valuable for all children, parents and staff, as well as being necessary to support more complex challenging children. The concepts introduced in the training are not revolutionary – many staff routinely implement these interventions as they are part of our common knowledge around parenting. However, this study suggests that by having an articulated conceptual framework to support this work, staff feel more confident in meeting the child's and parent's needs.

There is growing awareness of these concerns and developments and it is important that children's services allow a paradigm shift to enable greater resources to be invested in the early years. It is important to recognise that staff require ongoing training and support to deal with complex demanding relationships. By truly valuing partnership working with parents and understanding that even very young children may have very complex psychological needs and addressing them at the earliest possible opportunity, we can impact on the health inequality gradient (see Chapter 1).

The child-minding workforce is well placed to provide high quality care to vulnerable children; it is important that further research captures their views on this work and learns from their extensive experience. It is hoped that in emphasising the importance of attunement and regulation for all relationships, early years systems will develop to not only meet the child and parent's needs in this area but recognise the importance of these processes for all staff who support families with complex needs to enable them to stay healthily involved, compassionate and professional within this work.

Notes

1   The Department for Children, Schools and Families (DCSF) was a department of the UK Government, between 2007 and 2010.
2   Ofsted: Office for Standards in Education, Children's Services and Skills for England. Amongst other services Ofsted inspects or regulates child-minding, child day care and children's centres.

References

Adair, D. (2009) *Changing Concepts of Vulnerability. Abstract from an Independent Study*. York: City of York Council.

Barlow, J., McMillan, A. S., Kirkpatrick, S., Ghate, D., Barnes, J. and Smith, M. (2010) Health-led interventions in the early years to enhance infant and maternal mental health: a review of reviews. *Child and Adolescent Mental Health* 15, 4: 178–185.

Bayer, J. K., Hiscock, H., Morton-Allen, E., Ukoumunne, O. C. and Wake, M. (2007) Prevention of mental health problems: rationale for a universal approach. *Archives of Disease in Childhood* 92: 34–38 doi:10.1136/adc.2006.100776.

Booth, P. and Jenberg, A. (2010) *Theraplay: Helping Parents and Children Build Better Relationships through Attachment-Based Play*. San Francisco, CA: Wiley.

Child Psychotherapy Trust (2002) *An Infant Mental Health Service: The Importance of the Early Years and Evidence-Based Practice*. Online at: http://understandingchildhood.net/documents/32IMHreport.pdf Accessed September 2013.

Crittenden, P. (2013) *Dynamic Maturation Model of Attachment*. Online at: http://www.patcrittenden.com/include/dmm_model.htm Accessed September 2013.

Department for Education (2012) *Early Education and Childcare: Statutory Guidance for Local Authorities*. Online at: http://www.education.gov.uk/aboutdfe/statutory/g00209650/code-of-practice-for-las Accessed September 2013.

Department for Education and Department of Health (2011) *Supporting Families in the Foundation Years*. Online at: https://www.gov.uk/government/publications/supporting-families-in-the-foundation-years Accessed September 2013.

Department of Health (2009) *Healthy Child Programme: Pregnancy and the First 5 Years of Life*. Online at: https://www.gov.uk/government/publications/healthy-child-programme-pregnancy-and-the-first-5-years-of-life Accessed August 2013.

Gerhardt, S. (2004) *Why Love Matters: How Affection Shapes a Baby's Brain.* London: Routledge.

Heckman, J. J. (2011) The economics of inequality: the value of early childhood education. *American Educator* 35, 1: 31–47.

Heckman, J. J. (2000) 'The real question is how to use the available funds wisely. The best evidence supports the policy prescription: Invest in the Very Young'. Ounce of Prevention Fund and University of Chicago. Online at: http://www.ounceofprevention.org/news/pdfs/heckmaninvestinveryyoung.pdf Accessed September 2013.

Hughes, D. A. and Baylin, J. (2012) *Brain-Based Parenting.* New York: Norton.

Karr-Morse, R. and Wiley, M. S. (2012) *Scared Sick: The Role of Childhood Trauma in Adult Disease.* New York: Basic Books.

Kennedy, I. (2010) *Getting It Right for Children and Young People: Overcoming Cultural Barriers in the NHS so as to Meet Their Needs.* Online at: https://www.gov.uk/government/uploads/system/uploads/attachment_data/file/216282/dh_119446.pdf Accessed September 2013.

NSPCC (2011) *Child Abuse and Neglect in the UK Today. NSPCC Research.* Online at: http://www.nspcc.org.uk/Inform/research/findings/child_abuse_neglect_research_PDF_wdf84181.pdf Accessed September 2013.

Perry, B. (2004) *Understanding Traumatised and Maltreated Children: The Core Concepts.* Child trauma academy. Online at: http://www.lfcc.on.ca/Perry_Core_Concepts_Violence_and_Childhood.pdf Accessed September 2013.

Perry, B. (2002) *Six Core Strengths for Healthy Child Development.* Online at: http://www.lfcc.on.ca/Perry_Six_Core_Strengths.pdf Accessed September 2013.

Shonkoff, J. D. and Garner, A. S. (2011) The lifelong effects of early childhood adversity and toxic stress. *Pediatrics* 129, 1, 2012, pp. 2011–2663 doi: 10.1542/peds.

Shonkoff, J. D. and Phillips, D. A. (eds) (2000) *From Neurons to Neighbourhoods: The Science of Early Childhood Development.* Washington, DC: National Academy Press.

Solihull Primary Care Trust (2004) *The Solihull Approach Resource Pack: The First Five Years.* Solihull Primary Care Trust and University of Central England in Birmingham.

WAVE Trust and Department for Education (2013a) *Invited Response to Supporting Families in the Foundation Years.* Online at: http://www.wavetrust.org/key-publications/reports/conception-to-age-2 Accessed September 2013.

WAVE Trust and Department for Education (2013b) *Conception to Age 2 – The Age of Opportunity: Addendum to the Government's Vision for the Foundation Years: 'Supporting Families in the Foundation Years'.* Online at: http://www.inspiredbybabies.org.uk/Page8FacilitatorsUpdatesresources/Conception%20-2%20An%20age%20of%20opportunity%20.pdf Accessed September 2013.

Zeedyck M. S. (2011) *What About the Children? Why My Buggy Matter: Neuroscience on the Street.* Online at: http://suzannezeedyk.com/content/uploads/2011/03/why-my-buggy-matters-2011_1.pdf Accessed September 2013.

5

ADDRESSING HEALTH INEQUALITIES FOR MOTHERS AND BABIES IN PRISON

Findings from a consultation exercise

Katherine Albertson, Caroline O'Keeffe, Catherine Burke, Georgina Lessing-Turner and Mary Renfrew

Introduction

Current public health discourse includes concepts such as fairness, social justice and equity of access to health services. These concepts are examined here within the findings of a small consultation project, conducted in the UK in 2010, concerning health provision to mothers and babies in prison in the UK. The project links directly to the policy objective in the *Fair Society, Healthy Lives* report (Marmot 2010) to give every child the best start in life by ensuring high quality services are utilised to reduce inequalities in early child development. Further clear links to Marmot's policy are evident, including the recommendation to give priority to pre- and post-natal interventions that reduce adverse outcomes of pregnancy and infancy. The consultation reported here employed a range of qualitative consultation methods with health and prison staff to capture a real-world view of potential positive outcomes and the challenges of providing services to this population. Including women with experience of this service provision unfortunately proved impossible due to unrealistic project and prison service permission timescales.

Underpinning theory and policy: what we know about mothers and babies in prison

Women in prison are disproportionally likely to be poor, from socially deprived demographic backgrounds, have experience of unemployment, mental illness and be victims of abuse (Corston 2007; Social Exclusion Unit 2002). These are risk factors which are likely to result in impaired physical, social and emotional wellbeing as well as adverse short, medium and long term health outcomes (Field 2010; Marmot 2010). Indeed, mothers in prison are more likely than the general population to experience perinatal and maternal mortality and morbidity, and to suffer separation from their children and result-ant distress (Birmingham et al. 2006; Gregoire et al., 2010; Siefert and Pimott, 2001). In terms of changes in public health discourse and the life course model outlined in Chapter

1 of this book, the concepts of a health divide and social justice are clear when examining this small, but vulnerable, population. The Government's recent Green Paper: 'Breaking the Cycle' (Ministry of Justice 2010) not only stresses the importance of addressing offender health needs as part of the rehabilitation revolution, but highlights health as an important pathway to reduce reoffending.

There is broad consensus that wherever possible mothers with children should, in the first instance, be kept out of custody (e.g. Children's Commissioner for England 2008; Corston 2007). Where custody is unavoidable, however, residence on a Mother and Baby Unit (MBU) can provide an opportunity for improving the health and wellbeing of mothers and babies who would not normally access conventional health services outside prison, and who may be motivated to make changes for the sake of their babies' wellbeing (Edge 2006). An MBU in prison is designated living accommodation unit within existing women's or mixed gender prisons.

At the time of writing, there are seven MBU units in the UK, with 77 places in total. To contextualise, most countries in the European Union (EU) have some MBU provision, but this is varied in scope (with some countries only having access to a single MBU). Eight countries have no provision at all (Quaker Council for European Affairs 2007: 48). In 2007, the UK was reported as having the highest number of MBU places available in the EU and in this sense the UK can be seen as leading the way in developing MBU provision (see Alejos 2005).

MBUs in the UK are designed 'to reflect society's normal assumption that the best place for a young child is with his or her parent' (Prison Service Instruction 54/2011). A sentenced mother with a child under 18 months old can apply to have their child in prison with them; however some MBUs can only accept children up to 9 months. For mothers sentenced to custody of 18 months or over, arrangements are normally made for their children to be cared for outside prison (Prison Service Website 2012). To contextualise, in the EU the age children are allowed to stay in prison with their mother ranges from not being allowed in prison at all in Norway to being with their mother for up to four years old in Latvia (Quaker Council for European Affairs 2007: 51).

As the introductory chapters of this book summarise, the multitude of social factors at the root of health inequalities 'should be of concern to policy makers in every sector, not solely those involved in health policy' (Marmot 2005: 1099). Given the extreme disadvantage of mothers and babies in prison, it is clear that a 'joined-up' approach to addressing the health care needs of this small but extremely vulnerable group would be beneficial. There are significant challenges in effective co-ordination of and liaison between community health, prison, social and related services involved in delivering healthcare to childbearing women in prison (Edge 2006). Prison staff, probation officers and social workers may not have adequate knowledge of maternal and infant care whilst generic community health staff may not understand the constraints of the criminal justice system. Women may also be imprisoned at a distance from their immediate family and be without a social or family support network. The criminal justice system imposes non-negotiable constraints on communication and movement, without particular regard for the individual needs of a woman who may be pregnant, newly delivered or lactating. As a result, women in the criminal justice system are more likely to book late for antenatal care, receive minimal antenatal education, not receive adequate food and nutritional advice during pregnancy and postpartum, be without the support of a family member during labour and birth, have a premature or small-for-dates baby, decide to formula feed and be separated from their baby soon after birth (Edge 2006). In combination, these factors are highlighted as being key to positive health and wellbeing in the social model of health (Whitehead 1987). In this particular population, these factors may have a substantive impact on women's own physical and mental health, the nutrition, health and development of their babies, and on the appropriate development of attachment, parenting skills, and stable family relationships following release from prison.

The significance of pre-birth and early years in the life trajectory of children is outlined in Marmot's (2010) framework for action and the objective of 'giving every child the best start in life' is of the highest priority. He also states that disadvantage starts prior to birth and accumulates over the life course. Therefore, it is counter-intuitive to address the needs of a child's pre-birth and early years in isolation from her/his mother's needs. Further, important recent findings based on the Millennium Cohort Study show that early maternal health and wellbeing and maternal depression are both strong predictors of child health at age five, as well as child developmental and behavioural outcomes (Hobcraft and Kiernan 2010). Thus, there are important arguments for addressing these avoidable problems by providing care which optimises maternal physical and mental health, not only for the mother's sake, but also for that of her child's health and wellbeing in years to come. This is particularly pertinent for mothers in prison, who are more likely to experience poor health and poor maternal outcomes, as highlighted above, but are also a 'captive audience' for health promotion messages and interventions. Despite this, there is limited research evidence related to the specific health needs of childbearing women in prison and on ways of providing effective care which enables them to optimise their own life chances and those of their children.

The research and findings

The findings highlighted here are from a collaborative project between the Hallam Centre for Community Justice at Sheffield Hallam University and the Mother and Infant Research Unit at the University of York. This work involved conducting consultation activities with over 70 stakeholders, including focus groups with 15 health and prison staff involved in the delivery of mother and baby health services in MBUs in two female prisons in England. We interviewed five MBU Managers and utilised an online expert panel of 38 individuals with a range of expertise in women's health, maternity care, health inequalities and the criminal justice system. We hosted a multi-agency workshop event with 19 attendees which was particularly instrumental in identifying potential solutions to the challenges of delivering care to childbearing women in prison generally and in MBUs particularly. The seven topics for discussion used to guide the consultation exercises were: communication and partnership working, current pregnancy provision, the impact of prison setting on ability to deliver effective care, life on the MBU, mothering in the prison context, the separation process and processes around release from the MBU. The findings presented here focus on solutions to challenges identified.

Improving monitoring and data collection for childbearing women in prison

The number of pregnant and postpartum women in prison in the UK is not known as figures are not collated centrally. However, the Prison Reform Trust (2012) report that between April and June 2008, 49 women in prison gave birth.

Improved data collection regarding childbearing women in prison was identified as a starting point for enhancing healthcare provision. Such strategies would facilitate routinely collected national data, such as: the number of pregnant women in prison; the number of women in MBUs; the number of women with young babies who have not accessed/applied for an MBU place; birth weights of babies born to women in prison; and the numbers of stillbirths, miscarriages, terminations and infant/maternal mortality and morbidity. Such monitoring would enable policy makers to begin to identify the level and specific needs amongst this vulnerable cohort. In addition, participants recommended mapping existing delivery models of MBU provision in order to assess the effectiveness of different models of delivery, given that some MBUs are staffed by the prison, others by third sectors agencies and MBUs operate within both private and public sector prisons.

It was also suggested that identifying the availability of local community-based services would enable the linking up of community provision into each MBU and enhance the continued care for those women with babies being released in to the community. Longer term monitoring of child development and reoffending rates among MBU residents could also enable a comparative analysis of benefits with a control group, made up of those who have not accessed MBUs. These activities would ensure an assessment of the impact of MBU provision for both mothers and their children could be conducted. The collation of robust datasets would arguably enhance healthcare pathways for childbearing women in prison by providing an evidence base to underpin the commissioning of services and could also be utilised to facilitate a co-ordinated national approach to MBU provision.

A number of challenges were identified in adopting effecting monitoring systems within the prison service. These included: a lack of inter-institutional co-ordination amongst administrative staff, medical staff and operational prison staff; inconsistency between prisons around willingness and/or ability to collect such data; the risk of stigmatisation for individual prisons who may be identified as having especially negative outcomes; medical confidentiality and gaining consent from pregnant women and mothers in prison for such information to be disclosed; and the difficulties of 'keeping track' of the often highly transient prison population. For any national data collection strategy to be implemented it would be vital to garner support (and funding) from central government. Being explicit about why robust data is needed and how it will help both prisons and health services to better meet the needs of childbearing women and their babies will be crucial for obtaining such support. Strong leadership, for example, an identified monitoring lead, would also be crucial to ensure that health and criminal justice agencies work together to achieve a meaningful monitoring framework.

Improving multi-agency communication and collaboration around mothers in prison

Our research found that MBU Managers communicate well with each other (both informally and at quarterly meetings). Many prisons have excellent relationships with community midwives and health visitors. However, on an organisational level, communication and collaboration between prisons and healthcare systems were perceived to be poor. For example, one representative from a Community Midwifery Team reported there being no mechanism for informing midwives when pregnant women are admitted to prison or released into the community. The long delays in this information filtering through (often through court reports or word of mouth among colleagues) was felt to have a very negative impact on on-going antenatal care especially where pregnancies are high risk or where there are child protection concerns. Examples were also provided where more generic community health sector staff often had little experience of working with women who have come into contact with the criminal justice sector. This resulted in these staff having a lack of understanding of their patients' complex needs as well as little knowledge of risk assessment procedures and prison regime issues which may impact on their delivery of care to this cohort. Some consultation participants also reported limited engagement from certain key agencies, for example, hospitals and court staff who often remain uncommunicative at a more strategic level.

Participants reported that improving collaborative working among relevant agencies would require: investing in networking and information-sharing activities between prison and health staff; ensuring that clear, direct lines of communication were in place; developing multi-agency protocols which would guide the journey through the criminal justice system (community, prison, release and maintenance in the community post-release) for these vulnerable women and their babies. A key barrier to joined-up working was felt to be the insular nature of the prison service and the existence of a culture which does not facilitate the sharing of good practice and collaborative working practices with outside agencies. There was a perception that 'data protection arguments' between agencies could be prohibitive. There was perceived to be a lack of prioritisation of pregnant women and new mothers both within the prison service and also the health service which may impede efforts to work more collaboratively, particularly in these times of budget and staff cuts. Practical concerns regarding releasing 'hands-on' prison staff to attend networking events and also the fact that health agencies in the community are frequently at some geographical distance from prisons were also raised as challenges.

Despite these various barriers, numerous ways of enhancing communication and networking were suggested. Some of these relate specifically to procedures, for example, the development of information-sharing protocols between prisons and healthcare agencies, midwives and local safeguarding teams to ensure on-going antenatal care and input from all appropriate agencies; a set of mandatory national guidelines for the health provision of mothers in prison which ensure consistency and equity across the female prison estate and into the community. Others relate to ensuring appropriate personnel are in place to support collaborative working (e.g. identification of a link person with responsibility for this client group in each key agency) and obtaining 'buy in' from strategic level criminal justice and health staff. Such developments would assist in providing a more 'joined-up' care pathway for childbearing women and babies coming into contact with the criminal justice system.

Developing the potential of childbearing women in prison: examples of good practice

Participants discussed how childbearing women in prison (especially those in MBUs) are a receptive audience for personal development opportunities and health promotion messages. All participants were committed to enhancing these opportunities. During this consultation exercise, activities were identified that enable mothers in prison to understand and respond to their babies' needs. Just a few examples include: 'Birth Companion Parenting Groups' at HMP Holloway and Rainsbrook Secure Training Centre, which is also attended by fathers; the Anna Freud 'New Beginnings' course, based on the principles of 'attachment theory' (Baradon et al. 2008); 'Stay and Play' sessions at HMP Askham Grange, attended as part of sentence planning to encourage bonding between mother and child; and the social enterprise company, 'Little Angels' breastfeeding support at HMP New Hall (Albertson et al. 2012).

There was broad consensus that such capacity-building activities and courses recognising parenthood education should be part of their prison programme. It was felt that this should be incorporated nationally into overall sentence planning for mothers to provide equity of care by mirroring (as far as possible) the positive parenting experience of mothers in the community. Engaging the wider family and support networks of mothers and babies in prison with as many of these activities as possible was also seen as effective practice.

Mothers with babies in MBUs generally have to leave them during the day at a very young age, normally six weeks after giving birth, to engage with sentence-planning activities. This may have a detrimental impact upon their ability to attend antenatal and/ or parenting classes, which they often have to attend in their 'free' time. Some mothers may be due to give birth on arrival in prison and may not have time to complete a course; others may be moved at short notice resulting in a curtailed course attendance. The numbers of pregnant women in prison and mothers in MBUs fluctuate. There may not be sufficient numbers to make courses viable. The provision of education within prisons is not within the establishment's control, making it difficult to have any impact on the courses which are provided. Referring back to Marmot's policy recommendations regarding giving priority to pre- and postnatal interventions that reduce adverse outcomes of pregnancy and early infancy, one can see that there are a number of significant challenges that make this objective more complex in practice.

Consultation participants overwhelmingly supported the implementation of activities which could enhance the personal development of mothers in prison, especially those which enable them to parent effectively. Mechanisms for ensuring the provision of parenting support for these mothers were suggested as follows: ring-fenced budgets for commissioning ante- and postnatal services; commissioning service providers that can demonstrate their effectiveness; building activities into the sentence planning of all mothers and pregnant prisoners and ensuring there is support in place for release (e.g. through the involvement of family members, Prison Family Workers, Visitor Centre staff and Women's Centres).

Application to policy and practice

Mothers in prison, particularly those who reside in MBUs, are a small but extremely vulnerable group. However, the impact on the care and services they require is disproportionately large, with significant resources spent on health, development, education and social services over many years resulting from ill health, delayed development and family disruption (Corston 2007). Whilst in prison, they are a 'captive audience' for health promotion and intervention which may vastly improve the health and wellbeing of their children in both the short and long term, issues which link directly to Marmot's policy objectives. This is particularly pertinent given the evidence borne out of desistance[1] literature that significant life transitions can assist the rejection of offending lifestyles (Kreager et al. 2010).

The results of this consultation offer a mixed picture of provision for the health and wellbeing of this cohort. The lack of robust evidence for developing policy and practice is problematic, particularly given the vulnerability of MBU populations to health inequalities later in life. The consultation revealed a high level of experience, expertise and enthusiasm among both prison and health sector staff to support these mothers and their babies during this crucial life stage. However, despite considerable evidence of good practice there is scant indication of a more strategic approach to practice. The point at which health and prison services interact can be problematic due to a range of factors including cultures of working and a lack of understanding of the organisational constraints within which other agencies involved work. Gaps in communication at the point of entry into prison and on release are particularly problematic. Difficulties exist with implementing antenatal and parenting support within the confines of a prison setting where sentence-planning activities may take priority especially at a time when funding is so scarce.

This consultation has begun to take some tentative steps towards developing an agenda for working with mothers and babies in the criminal justice system in general and in MBUs in particular. Significantly, this consultation has identified an active interest, commitment, and common purpose across multiple agencies to improve the situation of mothers of young children coming into contact with the criminal justice system in the UK. Although good practice examples exist internationally and examining these could be beneficial (see Alejos 2005), the UK could potentially lead the way in developing high quality services based on these policy recommendations. These policy developments could ultimately feed into the progression of international standardisation practices for mothers and babies in prison currently being called for (see for example, Omolara Ojeah 2010).

This consultation has shown the value of tapping into the wealth of experience of both prison and health practitioners in this field, as to highlighting realistic proposals to assist in ensuring the highest standards of care are provided for this vulnerable population. It also indicates how mixed and varied research methods that capture different perspectives can help map service need, service provision and priorities for the future. Using evidence that explores lay perspectives is important for public health in the future (see Chapter 1 of this book). However, an unavoidable omission here was the voices of the very women with experience of being in prison with their babies. This is a key recommendation for further research.

Note

1   The process by which people stop offending.

References

Albertson, K. E., O'Keeffe, C., Lessing-Turner, G., Burke, C. and Renfrew, M. J. (2012) *Tackling Health Inequalities through Developing Evidence-Based Policy and Practice with Childbearing Women in Prison: A Consultation.* Hallam Centre for Community Justice, Sheffield Hallam University, May 2012. Online at: http://www.cjp.org.uk/publications/tackling-health-inequalities/ Accessed September 2013.

Alejos, M. (2005) *Babies and Small Children Residing in Prisons.* Quaker United Nations Office, March 2005. Online at: http://quno.org/geneva/pdf/200503Babies-Small-Children-in-Prisons-English.pdf Accessed September 2013.

Baradon, T., Fonagy, P., Bland, K., Lenard, K. and Sleed, M. (2008) New Beginnings: an experience-based programme addressing the attachment relationship between mothers and their babies in prisons. *Journal of Child Psychotherapy* 34, 2: 240–258.

Birmingham, L., Coulson, D., Mullee, M., Kamal, M. and Gregoire, A. (2006) The mental health of women in prison mother and baby units. *The Journal of Forensic Psychiatry and Psychology* 17, 3: 393–404.

Children's Commissioner for England (2008) *The 11 Million Report: Prison Mother and Baby Units: Do They Meet the Best Interest of the Child?* Online at: http://www.prisonersfamilies.org.uk/uploadedFiles/2010_Policy/Prison_Mother_and_Baby_Units.pdf Accessed September 2013.

Corston, J. (2007) *The Corston Report: A Review of Women with Particular Vulnerabilities in the Criminal Justice System.* London: Home Office, 2007.

Edge, D. (2006) *Perinatal Healthcare in Prison: A Scoping Review of Policy and Provision.* The Prison Health Research Network, Department of Health. Online at: http://www.ohrn.nhs.uk/resource/Research/PCSysRevPerinatal.pdf Accessed September 2013.

Field, F. (2010) *The Foundation Years: Preventing Poor Children Becoming Poor Adults. The Report of the Independent Review of Poverty and Life Chances.* Online at: http://dera.ioe.ac.uk/14156/1/poverty-report.pdf Accessed September 2013.

Gregoire, A., Dolan, R., Birmingham, L., Mullee, M. and Coulson, D. (2010) The mental health and treatment needs of imprisoned mothers of young children. *Journal of Psychiatry and Psychology* 21, 3: 378–392.

Hobcraft, J. N. and Kiernan, K. E. (2010) *Predictive Factors from Age 3 and Infancy for Poor Child Outcomes at Age 5 relating to Children's Development, Behaviour and Health: Evidence from the Millennium Cohort Study, University of York.* Online at: http://www.york.ac.uk/iee/assets/HobcraftKiernan2010PredictiveFactorsChildrensDevelopmentMillenniumCohort.pdf Accessed September 2013.

Kreager, D. A., Matsueda, R. L. and Erosheva, E. A. (2010) Motherhood and criminal desistance in disadvantaged neighbourhoods. *Criminology* 48, 1: 221–258.

Marmot, M. (2005) Social determinants of health inequalities. *Lancet* 365, 9464: 1099–1104.

Marmot, M. (2010) *Fair Society, Healthy Lives: Strategic Review of Health Inequalities in England post 2010*. Online at: http://webarchive.nationalarchives.gov.uk/+/www.dh.gov.uk/en/Publichealth/Healthinequalities/DH_094770 Accessed September 2013.

Ministry of Justice (2010) *Breaking the Cycle: Effective Punishment, Rehabilitation and Sentencing of Offenders*. Online at: http://sentencing.justice.gov.uk/?id=5&id2=14 Accessed September 2013.

Omolara Ojeah, E. (2010) *Consolidating International Standards Rules for Mothers with Babies in Prison*. Paper presented to the Centre for Prison Studies, Mothers and Babies in Prison Conference 2010 at Salford University. Online at: http://www.salford.ac.uk/__data/assets/pdf_file/0006/129228/CONSOLIDATING_INTERNATIONAL_STANDARD_RULES_FOR_MOTHERS.pdf Accessed September 2013.

Prison Reform Trust (2012) *Women in Prison*. Online at: http://www.prisonreformtrust.org.uk/Portals/0/Documents/Women's%20briefing%20March12.pdf Accessed September 2013.

Prison Service Instruction 54/2011: Section 1.1. Mother and Baby Units Online at: https://www.google.co.uk/webhp?source=search_app&gws_rd=cr&ei=mhw8UrTjHcy20wX7uYCYDw#q=+Prison+Service+Instruction+54%2F2011%3A+Section+1.1. Accessed September 2013.

Prison Service Web site (2012) *Pregnancy and Childcare in Prison*. Online at: https://www.gov.uk/life-in-prison/pregnancy-and-childcare-in-prison. Accessed September 2013.

Quaker Council for European Affairs (2007) *A Review of the Conditions in Member States of the Council of Europe, Report*. Online at: http://www.qcea.org/wp-content/uploads/2011/04/rprt-wip1-main-en-feb-2007.pdf Accessed September 2013.

Siefert, K. and Pimott, S. (2001) Improving pregnancy outcomes during imprisonment: a model residential care program. *Social Work* 46, 2: 125–134.

Social Exclusion Unit (2002) *Reducing Re-offending by Ex-prisoners*. Online at: http://www.social-finance.org.uk/sib/guides/social-exclusion-taskforce-reducing-re-offending-ex-prisoners Accessed September 2013.

Whitehead, M. (1987) *Inequalities in Health in the 1980s*. Online at: http://www.dur.ac.uk/publichealth.library/HDA_archive/5172%20-%2054007000092122%20-%20WHITE-HEAD%20-%20THE%20HEALTH%20DIVIDE.pdf Accessed September 2013.

6

CHILDREN IN FULL-TIME EDUCATION (AGES 5–16)

Chris Bentley

Introduction

The Marmot Review Policy Objective B states the need to 'Enable all children, young people and adults to maximise their capabilities and have control over their lives'. The recommendations within that objective place significant weight on the time children spend in full-time education. Recommendations therefore include direction to:

1. Extend the role of schools in supporting families and communities and taking a 'whole child' approach to education;
2. Have consistent implementation of the full range of extended services in and around schools;
3. Develop the school-based workforce to build their skills in working across school-home boundaries and addressing social and emotional development, physical and mental health and well-being.

As part of this approach, schools should be providing social, behavioural, psychiatric and other special needs support progressively across the social gradient (Marmot Review 2010: 182–183). Both chapters in this section explore the current application of these principles, and future scope for change, around issues related to developing sexuality and supporting the health and wellbeing of young people.

Promoting positive sexuality and sexual health for young people in full-time education

Sex and relationships education (SRE) in schools and colleges should be an important tranche of the Marmot Review recommendations, both in enabling young people to maximise their capabilities and have control over their lives, and also strengthening the role and impact of ill health prevention. The emphasis on relationships, skills and values distinguishes SRE from more biologically orientated sex education. It represents that part of education that enables children 'to develop their personalities, talents and abilities, to build resilience, self-esteem, and to live a full and satisfying life' (Marmot Review: 104). In relation to this development of self, it will be important to consider respect for, and the rights of others.

Julia Hirst, in Chapter 7, establishes the importance of the intervention SRE, which she then explores in relation to theory and policy, but also by grounding the theory in a piece of detailed formal research with a number of young people of school age. It is fair to say that the content of the interviews, and the language used in the discussion, seem a very long way from the range of policy documents reviewed. This suggests there is some distance to go in order to bridge the gap between theoretical and practical needs in this area.

In relation to the possibilities of delivering population level change either for 'supporting young people to maximise their capabilities in negotiating positive outcomes' or ill health prevention, a number of major barriers currently exist within the Population Intervention Triangle (Chapter 2).

The first is in relation to population level intervention through legislation, regulation and healthy public policy. As Hirst states, 'SRE is a political issue, shrouded in ideological differences'. These differences can block the development of evidence-based policy. In 2007 the Department of Health commissioned NICE to produce guidance on Personal, Social, Health and Economic (PSHE) education focusing on sex and relationships, and alcohol education. The guidance was produced through the usual testing process, but prior to publication, the Department of Health (DH) suspended the commission. The full document was, however, submitted in evidence to the Department for Education's 2011 review of PSHE, and so is published in that form (NICE 2012). There are 12 recommendations, constituting a whole system programme for evidence-based practice, including:

- The provision of PSHE education
- Consultation with children and young people
- Planning and teaching
- External contributions and support
- Specifics on community-based education
- Training of educators

Such guidance might have produced the basis of consistent evidence-based practice, and it will be important to scrutinise what the Government's Department for Education makes of this input, and how the DH works with them to gain consistent approaches and leadership across the sectors.

However, in Chapter 7, Hirst also highlights another concern, which would, in any case, interrupt the systematic delivery through services, another apex of the Population Intervention Triangle. This involves the removal of a range of Free Schools and Academies from the legislative framework for SRE and sex education. They have been granted exemption under the terms of their funding agreements, and there is the danger/likelihood that personal or religious views can supersede guidance on best practice for SRE.

The danger posed by both of these factors is that implementation of best practice will continue to be patchy and variable, and the excellent population level outcomes achieved by Scandinavian countries and Holland, to which their version of SRE contributes, will continue to be unachievable evenly across the UK.

The emotional health and wellbeing of young people who identify as lesbian, gay, bisexual or transgender (LGBT)

Chapter 8 largely features the third apex of the Population Intervention Triangle, addressing as it does the need for intervention through (extended school) communities. Young people spend a large amount of their time in a school setting, and so the environment created can have a major impact on learned knowledge, beliefs and actions. Peer influences and pressure can be considerable in the shaping of developing individuals. This can be harnessed as a force for good, providing a supportive environment. However, dominant forces can emerge to create the opposite effect.

Eleanor Formby uses findings from a qualitative research project interviewing young people, staff and youth workers in South Yorkshire about knowledge, issues and approaches to LGBT and the ways this can impact on emotional wellbeing.

The results paint a predominantly discriminatory picture, documenting experiences, consequences and responses to homophobia and bullying. The negative experiences do not all emanate from peers, with teachers and youth workers in some cases colluding with a discriminatory culture. Policy and practice around the extended 'community' role of schools was seen to be influenced by the 'service' component of SRE, which was largely seen as institutionalising heterosexism and homophobia.

Such learned cultural roles obviously do not develop in isolation in the school environment, with outside-school influences such as the media, including social media, and pornography, for example, being predominant. However, as Hirst rehearses in her chapter, schools and colleges can offer a 'boundaried setting' that reaches a majority of young people who want education and support to help them protect and have greater control over their lives in relation to their sexual and emotional health and relationships. From a population health perspective, the question is how can this potential be more systematically capitalised upon in both the formal and 'extended school' settings?

Some positive practice is identified. Valued support offered by an LGBT-specific youth service included a safe environment for free discussion, and facilitated access to specialist and peer support. There is discussion about approaches which focus more on victims of homophobic bullying, with counselling support for example, or on the perpetrators, with a 'zero tolerance' approach. However, a fine line is identified between driving attitudes underground and favouring open debate. The research establishes that young people would prefer to see a far greater inclusion of LGBT identities within mainstreaming schooling and youth work practice, rather than a focus on tackling bullying or supporting individual LGBT young people on an incident basis.

Gaining consistent positive approaches within all schools on these critical issues for young people, as they develop their skills for life, will be important for the population as a whole. It will also be critical for sustaining emotional wellbeing at this critical transitional period of young people's lives. However, this is likely to remain patchy and variable without some central oversight, and particularly while increasing numbers of schools are allowed to opt out of, or fail to implement, guidance.

References

Marmot Review (2010) *Fair Society, Healthy Lives*. London: The Marmot Review.
NICE (2012) *PSHE: NICE Response to DfE Review of PSHE Education*. London: NICE.

7

PROMOTING POSITIVE SEXUALITIES, RELATIONSHIPS AND SEXUAL HEALTH FOR YOUNG PEOPLE IN EDUCATIONAL SETTINGS

Julia Hirst

Introduction

Educational settings provide ideal sites for learning about sexualities, relationships and sexual health (UNESCO 2009). This does not mean that young people are guaranteed to receive the type of input they would like (Hirst 2008); nor does it mean that family, peers, television, digital media, pornography and accessible sexual health services are unimportant in shaping sexual understanding and developing life skills (Marston and King 2006). What it does mean is that schools and colleges, in particular, offer a boundaried setting that reaches a majority of young people who want education and support to help them protect and have greater control over their lives in relation to their sexual and emotional health and relationships. However, this opportunity is often not capitalised upon in the UK and countries where inadequate provision enhances susceptibility to exploitation, coercion, unplanned pregnancy and sexually transmitted infections, including HIV (Sidibé 2009). A significant factor is that sex and relationships education (SRE) is still regarded as controversial, with a lack of agreement on content, approaches and policy that could support more collective endeavours to increase the contribution it could make to health outcomes.

The aim of this chapter is to outline some aspects of sexual health and SRE and the role that schools and colleges might play in meeting the Marmot objectives of strengthening the role and impact of ill health prevention and enabling young people to maximise their capabilities and have control over their lives. After defining key terms, the chapter will briefly summarise the adversarial nature of SRE and its current policy status. Policy developments relate mainly to the UK, though issues raised have direct relevance for contexts where SRE is similarly disputed. Attention then turns to qualitative insights from young people that highlight some of the weaknesses in provision. Finally, the implications for practice and ways forward are considered.

Underpinning theory and policy

Defining sex education, SRE and sexual health

Sex education refers to input focusing largely on puberty, reproduction and sexually transmitted infections (STIs). In many countries, this forms part of the science curriculum. It is compulsory in the UK. SRE is more comprehensive and includes lifelong learning about sexuality, emotions, relationships, sexual health and wellbeing.

The emphasis on relationships, skills and values distinguishes SRE from more biologically oriented *sex education* (Sex Education Forum [SEF] 2011). SRE is not part of the statutory curriculum.

Biomedical models (see Chapter 1) tend to construct sexual health negatively in emphasising the individual and preventing STIs and unplanned pregnancy, despite the World Health Organisation's holistic definition (WHO [unofficial] 2002). In practice, where notions of SRE and sexual health are applied in relation to the WHO approach, the prevention of unplanned pregnancy and diseases remains prominent but the acquisition of knowledge and skills is promoted in relation to broader issues of sexual self-efficacy, relationships, responsible choices, safety, potential for pleasure, and respect for rights. Together with youth-friendly sexual health services, such approaches can support young people to maximise their capabilities in negotiating positive outcomes, exercising control and protecting their sexual health (Center for Reproductive Rights 2008). International research (Kirby 2007) including poorer countries (Boyce et al. 2007) and reviews of reviews (Downing et al. 2006) suggests that if Marmot objectives are to be realised, these broader concepts of SRE and sexual health should be integral to education and health services provision.

International literature underlines some excellent practice. Conspicuously, in the Netherlands, Denmark and Sweden, this correlates with the lowest rates for teenage pregnancy, abortions, STIs, later age of sexual debut and inter-relationship violence (see Ingham and Hirst 2010). MacDonald's (2009) UK review noted pockets of excellent practice but little evidence that comprehensive SRE occurs in more than a minority of schools. Similar conclusions emerged from UNESCO's (2009) review of global evidence. Though socio-cultural and economic differences must be acknowledged, it is notable that in contexts adopting sex-positive, comprehensive approaches, SRE is largely uncontroversial and unopposed. In contrast, the UK and Anglophone countries such as Australia, New Zealand and numerous other countries are reluctant to adopt comprehensive models of sexual health and SRE because of disputes that have endured the last half-century. The contribution this makes to poorer sexual health outcomes, earlier sexual debut, sexual coercion (Wellings et al. 2001) and violence within relationships is becoming increasingly recognised (Beasley 2008).

Debates and politics on SRE – solution or problem for public health outcomes?

Second World War policy-makers attempted to improve sex education in British schools in recognition of the increasing incidence of STIs (Hampshire and Lewis 2004). Hostilities were stirred, however, by the 'permissiveness' of the 1960s and a furore was born that has conflated sex education with opposition to reform, and the allegation that sex education has the potential to corrupt young people (Jackson 1996). Controversies and disagreements have endured for the ensuing half-century, with opponents seeing sex education as a *problem* and proponents as a *solution* to public health problems (see Goldman 2008).

Though SRE remains non-compulsory in all schools, it can be contained within non-statutory Personal, Social and Health Education (PSHE). The Education Act (1996) and the Learning and Skills Act (2000) provide the legislative framework for SRE and sex education but Free Schools and Academies were granted exemptions under the terms of their funding agreements in 2010 (SEF 2011). This means that though there must be regard for SRE guidance, in contrast to other maintained schools there is no requirement for an up-to-date policy and SRE can be taught in line with the school's religious ethos.

The model for Free Schools and Academies has potential to reduce balanced input on SRE, promote abstinence education for which there is no reliable evidence of positive outcomes (Avert 2012; Santelli et al. 2006) and inheres a heteronormativity in the emphasis on marriage between women and men and the importance of family life (SEF 2011: 3) that could undermine the right to non-discriminatory education for lesbian, gay, bisexual and trans (LGBT) young people (see further discussion in Formby's chapter). Notions of social justice, fairness and control (see Chapter 1) as mechanisms that can contribute to preventing ill health and enabling young people to maximise their capabilities and have control over their lives could be challenged for some young people.

In sum, content and approaches are likely to remain *ad hoc* and divide opinion for the foreseeable future. Discussion moves now to research evidence that offers a reminder of some of the reasons for making SRE a statutory part of the curriculum and questioning the reliance on science-based sex education.

The research approach and findings

This research study explores socialising, sexual practices and SRE among 15–16-year-old students from a school in a city in England. A qualitative mixed methodology was used to elicit views and develop understanding of experiences from the standpoint of participants' everyday lives, in their own words. Data cited below offer insight into a selection of these issues with a focus on the disjunction between sexual and relationships experiences and the SRE[1] they received. Findings point to issues young people regard as salient to more meaningful input and complement epidemiological data, such as that on age of sexual debut, rates of unprotected sex, conceptions, abortions and STIs.

Participants comprised 11 young women and four young men. All described themselves as straight though commented on experiences of gay peers. Ethnicities included African-Caribbean, Irish, Pakistani, Somali and white, and all described themselves as 'working class' and lived in relatively deprived neighbourhoods. Data collection occurred on school premises, during lunchtime and after classes. The mixed method approach involved a series of four focus groups comprising all 15 participants (45–60 minutes), three small group interviews (two single gender and one mixed) and five individual interviews (60–90 minutes). Interviews were akin to conversations and provided ample space for privileging the participants' voices.

While the study is small, the data are substantiated by a significant body of other evidence (see Ingham and Hirst 2010, for overview). In addition, the number of interviews (between three and seven) with each participant produced in-depth data, and the mixed methods allowed data to be triangulated and checked for authenticity. Over time, participants added detail, asked questions and queried disclosures made in previous encounters. This offered further opportunities for corroboration and validity checks. As the Leeds Declaration (Long 1993) recommends, such reflexive, qualitative approaches are important in prioritising lay people's views and understanding experiences as they relate to economic, social and political factors, as well as complementing findings from other disciplines and methodologies.

Findings are summarised in the third person and extracts from verbatim disclosures have been anonymised and attributed via pseudonyms.

Young people's perspectives

Poor sexual health is a complex issue and its relationship to wider inequalities cannot be understated. Nevertheless, there are aspects in traditional sex education (and its role in sexual health) that are more easily attended to. In summary they include: input is too late and does not match the realities of young people's experience; sexual behaviour is the focus and addressed in isolation from relationships and contexts; heterosexuality and vaginal penetration are privileged above other sexual identities and practices; there are too few opportunities for discussion and developing communication skills; emphasis is on the negative outcomes of sexual acts with minimum attention to the place of pleasure, agency, autonomy and self-esteem in effecting safer sexual practices; and the potential for manipulation, coercion and sexual violence is ignored. The analytic themes that follow make reference to a selection of these points.

Impact of context on sexual negotiations and subjectivity

A key finding was the differences between actual sexual experience and that offered in sex education. For example, sex was not a private act, nor restricted to indoor locations (e.g. bedrooms). Rather, it was intrinsic to their socialising. Furthermore, venues for sex rarely facilitated negotiation over its safety, insofar as encounters were furtive, often rushed and in the vicinity of others. For white and African-Caribbean males and females, all sexual activity had occurred outdoors, with friends nearby:

> Well it [sex] only happens on a Friday night at the park, when t'others [friends] are there [. . .]. Most of us have to be in by half past ten at latest . . . so it can be a bit rushed.
>
> *(Maisie)*

> I've always had my clothes on or most of 'em. I've never done it inside in a comfy warm bedroom or bed even, and I've been wet and freezing loads of times.
>
> *(Julie)*

Only Hanif and Javed (Pakistani males) had had sex indoors, in a one-roomed bedsit above Hanif's workplace (his part time job after school), but not in private:

> We [. . .] share the room, there's only one . . . so it's never . . . like . . . private. You just don't have big lights on . . . [we] share the room and the lasses know that.
>
> *(Hanif)*

Sex educators' disregard for the impact of context (be it lack of privacy, time, weather, etc.) on negotiating sexual safety was not lost on participants:

> Yeah, they [teachers] don't mention how cold it is when they're on about contraception . . . or, that you have to be quick 'cos you haven't got all the time in the world. It's not nice and relaxed like they [teachers] make out [suggest].
>
> *(Maisie)*

For young women, contrasts between settings for actual sexual activities and the idealised, romantic imagery that surrounds (some) school-based SRE contributed to inconsistencies in expectation and reality, sense of self and fears of condemnation:

> Yeah it's horrible really to think you have to get all mucky and get leaves on your bum [sex in the park]. It's nowt like you thought it were gonna be, like in films and sex education lessons.
>
> *(Josie)*

> Don't exactly make you feel good about yourself.
>
> *(Jo)*

> It's not just that we are doing it [having sex], it's that folk would go mad if they knew we did it in the park, and it's not exactly how you'd like it to be either or how you thought it would be.
>
> *(Maisie)*

Sexual negotiation is facilitated by confidence and positive sense of self (Hirst 2008) but involvement in 'public' sex diminishes the potential to achieve this.

Sexual repertoires and heterosexist norms

SRE is ostensibly concerned with delaying and/or promoting safer sexual behaviour and preventing ill health (Sex Education Forum 2011). For those already sexually active, useful education would include guidance on a range of safer sexual activities. But these young people experienced SRE that limited sexual behaviour, without exception, to vaginal penetration. This contrasts with the more extensive sexual repertoires disclosed by young people that included kissing (on lips, breasts, genitals), mutual masturbation (referred to as 'fondling', 'rubbing off' and 'fingering') and oral sex (referred to as 'gobbing off' and 'licking out'). These safer behaviours were more commonplace than is acknowledged by sex educators. Similarly, the range of sexual experiences between those with substantial or no experience was unacknowledged:

> It's like in sex education, you either have sex, as in, with a willy inside ya, or you don't. Well it's not true, there's all sorts goes on between that.
>
> *(Angela)*

By including this continuum, opportunities are created to promote safer non–penetrative sexual practices (which some were striving for) and is inclusive of same sex practices. Likewise, failure to do so can reinforce a sense of 'correctness' or legitimacy of vaginal penetration over other forms of sexual expression:

> There's nothing for me in sex education . . . I know all the stuff about how to have a baby but they don't tell us owt about other types of sex. It's stupid 'cos it makes you think you're maybe a bit weird 'cos you're not having *proper* sex.
>
> *(Julie; her emphasis)*

Heteronormativity is also exposed. The terms 'real sex', 'going all the way', 'doing it properly' and 'getting down to the basic thing' were used throughout, and were defined by interviewees as descriptions of vaginal penetration that could include ejaculation. These construct vaginal penetration with a penis as the assumed outcome of 'proper' or 'real' sexual activity. Respondents surmised that these norms for 'doing it properly' came from school–based input:

> Never thought about it before, but suppose it's what you get given in sex education.
>
> *(Jo)*

Television and magazines were acknowledged as having a potential influence but were not as significant as the views of teachers:

> Suppose they do influence you but when it comes from teachers it sort of has more . . . I dunno . . . importance.
>
> *(Josie)*

The heteronormative agenda also appears to exclude discussion of anal sex. Also, participants knew of 'friends' who had anal sex to prevent pregnancy:

> It's safer, can't get pregnant.
>
> *(Josie)*

> If ya haven't got any jonnies [condoms].
>
> *(Jo)*

No interviewee had considered STIs (including HIV) through unprotected anal sex and could not recall covering it in school.

Pleasure, agency and sexual autonomy

The absence of pleasure in young people's narratives has been highlighted for two decades (Fine 1988). Participants did not mention pleasure until specifically questioned, and went on to ask for advice on ways to enhance enjoyment. These requests offer optimism for female agency but also provided an opportunity to encourage safer practices such as mutual masturbation. However, subsequent disclosures illustrated that such opportunities are unlikely to occur naturally because of normative discourses and expectations of judgements:

> Why has pleasure not been mentioned before?
>
> *(JH)*
>
> Well, you're just not used to talking about it.
>
> *(Jo)*
>
> How are you meant to admit ya like it? Teachers would think you're a slag.
>
> *(Maisie)*

Fear of threats to reputation and the absence of pleasure are not the only factors that reinforce the omission of a discourse of pleasure particularly for women. SRE curricula fail to provide a usable vocabulary for articulating desire or pleasure, and also promote (perhaps not deliberately) ideologies of women as passive with little or no agency, or entitlement to pleasure, in the failure to speak of any sexual practice other than vaginal intercourse, and illustrate it with images of women submissively positioned under the man. This is unsurprising, as Evans notes: policy might promote safe sex or 'abstinence' from sex, but never 'pleasurable' sex (2006: 237).

Application to practice

Research cited in this chapter points to what matters for young people. The selected extracts aim to support practitioners in challenging biologically based sex education and making a case for a young person-centred, sex-positive approach. The key issues are discontinuing the emphasis on negative outcomes and instead promoting positive possibilities. In practice, this could mean acknowledging young people as sexual subjects with rights to agency, control and feeling good about themselves. Curriculum content would encourage a wider range of (safer) sexual repertoires, the ability to decide when and if they are ready for sex, and the potential for pleasure – irrespective of whether one is LGBT or straight. Institutionalised patriarchy, heterosexism and homophobia have to be challenged and addressed with conviction, together with undermining language or images which maintain women as passive or LGBT young people as 'abnormal' or invisible and heterosexual men as proactive sexual agents.

Skills development would address communication that encourages safer sexual practices, more egalitarian relationships and safeguarding by talking openly about coercion, abuse, sexual violence and hate crimes based on gender and sexualities. Young men have received less attention in this chapter but are acknowledged as equally important to negotiating safer sexual practices, control and equality in relationships. More evidence and theorising on young men, masculinities and pleasure are needed to support SRE programmes that address equality and mutual satisfaction in relationships

These are not all the reasons to promote positive SRE and good sexual heath. Others include critiquing mainstream pornography, preventing sexual dysfunction, and partnering SRE with accessible sexual health services. Hirst (2013, 2014) addresses this in more detail.

This chapter began by arguing that educational settings provide ideal sites for public health goals where the 'scaling-up' of programmes for illness prevention is facilitated through targeting a clearly defined population of young people. Whole-school approaches are routinely adopted for social and emotional aspects of learning, including anti-bullying and mental health issues (see Formby chapter), alcohol and drug education, physical activity and tackling obesity (see Aggleton et al. 2010). Schools and colleges host vaccination programmes for tuberculosis, human papillomavirus and health screening. Synergies between health and educational goals (Stewart-Brown 2006) also recognise the impact of social determinants in mediating educational disadvantage and poorer health (Brooks 2010). However, while a reciprocal relationship between health outcomes and education is largely uncontested and forms part of the health promoting and illness prevention role, this chapter has suggested that sexual health and education is more contentious with a lack of agreement on what young people need and should be offered, despite the fact that a majority of parents support SRE in educational contexts.

In the absence of government guidance on the statutory provision of SRE and freedoms afforded to free schools and academies to teach according to their school's ethos or priorities, perhaps one way forward is to stress the safeguarding agenda, since this is required by law. Yet, it is undeniable that persuading those who object to SRE on its merits is not easy. A recommended way forward is to work in a spirit of open partnership and dialogue with governors, parents, teachers, sexual health practitioners and young people in a process of listening to evidence, developing policy, planning content and approaches and routinely evaluating provision. Senior management and governors' support is crucial.

SRE is a political issue shrouded in ideological differences. Policies can lay down markers of how those in positions of responsibility in societies wish to treat their young people in relation to this most important area of health promotion and illness prevention.

Note

1   Though the school claimed to teach SRE, the content was more akin to biologically based sex education.

References

Aggleton, P., Dennison, C. and Warwick, I. (eds) (2010) *Promoting Health and Well-Being through Schools*. Abingdon: Routledge.

Avert (2012) *Abstinence and Sex Education.* Online at: http://www.avert.org/abstinence.htm Accessed September 2013.

Beasley, C. (2008) The challenge of pleasure: re-imagining sexuality and sexual health. *Health Sociology Review* 17, 2: 151–163.

Boyce, P., Huang Soo Lee, M., Jenkins, C., Mohamed, S., Overs, C., Paiva, V., Reid, E., Tan, M. and Aggleton, P. (2007) Putting sexuality (back) into HIV/AIDS: issues, theory and practice. *Global Public Health* 2, 1: 1–34.

Brooks, F. (2010) The health of children and young people. In P. Aggleton, C. Dennison and I. Warwick (eds) *Promoting Health and Well-Being through Schools.* Abingdon: Routledge, pp. 8–23.

Center for Reproductive Rights (2008) *An International Human Right: Sexuality for Adolescents in Schools.* New York: Center for Reproductive Rights.

Downing, J., Jones, L., Cook, P. A. and Bellis, M. A. (2006) *Prevention of Sexually Transmitted Infections (STIs): A Review of Reviews into the Effectiveness of Non-Clinical Interventions. Evidence Briefing Update.* Liverpool: Centre for Public Health, Liverpool John Moores University, for NICE.

Evans, D. (2006) 'We do not use the word "crisis" lightly . . .' Sexual health policy in the United Kingdom. *Policy Studies* 27, 3: 235–252.

Fine, M. (1988) Sexuality, schooling and adolescent females: the missing discourse of desire. *Harvard Educational Review* 58, 1: 29–53.

Goldman, J. (2008) Responding to parental objections to school sexuality education: A selection of 12 objections. *Sex Education* 8, 4: 415–438.

Hampshire, J. and Lewis, J. (2004) The ravages of permissiveness: Sex education and the permissive society. *Twentieth Century British History* 15, 3: 290–312.

Hirst, J. (2008) Developing sexual competence? Exploring strategies for the provision of effective sexualities and relationships education. *Sex Education* 8, 4: 399–413.

Hirst, J. (2013) 'It's got to be about enjoying yourself': young people, sexual pleasure, and sex and relationships education. *Sex Education* 13, 4: 423–436.

Hirst, J. (2014) 'Get some rhythm round the clitoris'. Addressing sexual pleasure in sexuality education in schools and other youth settings. In L. Allen, M. Rasmussen and K. Quinlivan (eds) *The Politics of Pleasure in Sexuality Education: Pleasure Bound.* New York: Routledge, pp. 35–56.

Ingham, R. and Hirst, J. (2010) Promoting sexual health. In P. Aggleton, C. Dennison and I. Warwick (eds) (pp. 99–118).

Jackson, S. (1996) *Childhood and Sexuality Revisited.* Basingstoke: Palgrave Macmillan.

Kirby, D. (2007) *Emerging Answers 2007: Research Findings on Programs to Reduce Teen Pregnancy and Sexually Transmitted Diseases.* Washington, DC: The National Campaign to Prevent Teen and Unplanned Pregnancy.

Long, A. F. (1993) *Understanding Health and Disease: Towards a Knowledge Base for Public Health Action.* Report of Workshop. Leeds: Nuffield Institute for Health.

Macdonald, A. (2009) *Independent Review of the Proposal to Make Personal, Social, Health and Economic Education (PSHE) Statutory.* London: Department for Children, Schools and Families.

Marston, C. and King, E. (2006) Factors that shape young people's sexual behaviour: a systematic review. *The Lancet* 368, 9547: 1581–1586.

Santelli, J. S., Ott, M. A., Lyon, M., Rogers, J., Summers, D. and Schleifer, R. (2006) Abstinence and abstinence-only education: a review of US policies and programs. *Journal of Adolescent Health* 38: 72–81.

Sex Education Forum (SEF) (2011) *Current Status of Sex and Relationships Education. SEF Briefing.* Online at: www.sexeducationforum.org.uk Accessed September 2013.

Sidibé, M. (2009) Foreword. *International Technical Guidance on Sexuality Education: An Evidence-informed Approach for Schools, Teachers and Health Educators, Volume 1: The Rationale for Sex Educators.* Paris: UNESCO.

Stewart-Brown, S. (2006) *What Is the Evidence on School Health Promotion in Improving Health or Preventing Disease and, Specifically, What Is the Effectiveness of the Health Promoting Schools Approach?* Copenhagen: WHO Regional Office for Europe. Health Evidence Network report. Online at: http://www.euro.who.int/document/e88185.pdf Accessed September 2013.

UNESCO (2009) *International Guidelines on Sexuality Education: An Evidence Informed Approach to Effective Sex, Relationships and HIV/STI Education.* Draft document. Paris: United Nations Educational, Scientific and Cultural Organisation.

Wellings, K., Nanchahal, W. et al. (2001). Sexual behaviour in Britain: early heterosexual experience. *The Lancet* 358, 9296: 1843–1850.

WHO (World Health Organisation) (2002) Sexual and Reproductive Health: Defining Sexual Health. Online at: http://www.who.int/reproductivehealth/publications/sexual_health/defining_sexual_health.pdf Accessed September 2013.

8

THE EMOTIONAL HEALTH AND WELLBEING OF YOUNG PEOPLE WHO IDENTIFY AS LESBIAN, GAY, BISEXUAL OR TRANS

Eleanor Formby

Introduction

This chapter examines evidence on the experiences of young lesbian, gay and bisexual (LGB) people, and the implications for their emotional health and wellbeing, based on a study of schools and youth work settings in South Yorkshire, England. In doing so, it also draws on other (inter)national evidence which indicates the transferability of the findings, and makes suggestions for future support for lesbian, gay, bisexual and trans (LGBT) young people. This is important in linking to three of the (2010) Marmot review objectives, concerning children, young people and adults maximising their capabilities and control over their lives; healthy sustainable places (e.g. schools and other youth-focused settings), and ill-health prevention.

The study explored barriers and facilitators to issues about (homo)sexuality, homophobia, (trans)gender identities and/or transphobia being included within schools and youth work settings. Whilst the research sought to include trans participants, unfortunately this material is limited, but care has been taken throughout to use the specific acronyms of 'LGB' or 'LGBT' where appropriate. Where implications for trans young people can be drawn out, these have been included.

The chapter begins with an outline of some of the existing evidence and practice in this field. This is followed by a brief description of the study methods, continuing with an overview of the study findings, and suggestions for practice.

Underpinning theory and policy: linking homophobia to public health

Recent years have seen a rise in interest in inequalities or prejudice facing LGBT people in the UK, and internationally. There is growing awareness, for instance, about health inequalities affecting LGBT communities in the UK (Fish 2007). Within this, particular attention is often paid to (poorer) mental health (King et al. 2008; McNeil et al. 2012).

For young LGBT people specifically, evidence from the UK and the US suggests higher incidences of self-harm, depression and/or attempted suicide compared with their heterosexual counterparts (McNamee et al. 2008; Robinson and Espelage 2011). They are also said to be more likely to suffer poorer physical health arising from higher incidences of alcohol, drug and/or tobacco use (Espelage et al. 2008; Rivers and Noret 2008), and may have poor experiences and/or a lack of access to appropriate healthcare or advice (Buston 2004; Formby 2011a). Caution is needed, however, to not over-state these 'risks', or portray LGBT people as inherently unhealthy and/or 'victimised'.

In line with a social model of health, a body of evidence suggests that LGBT health inequalities are linked to external contexts, as are numerous other health inequalities, and that we should examine and address homophobia in this light. Public health interventions could therefore acknowledge the lack of control some young people may have over their lives and related health outcomes; for example, young people may experience adverse reactions to their sexual and/or gender identities from parents and other family members (Formby 2012; Valentine et al. 2003). This may render the home environment hostile, and can lead to homelessness. Equally, schools and other settings where young people spend their time can be experienced as hostile and/or limiting young people's potential/capabilities. Existing research looking at LGB experiences of schooling in the UK, for instance, has identified discriminatory attitudes among some staff and broader invisibility of same-sex relationships and identities (Ellis and High 2004; Formby 2011b), as well as the prevalence of homophobic bullying and poor or inadequate responses from some schools (McNamee et al. 2008; Warwick et al. 2001). Studies have suggested that LGB young people are rarely included in the (formal) school curriculum because staff are uncomfortable, lacking confidence, or fearful about including LGB issues within their teaching, particularly regarding sex and relationships education (SRE) (DePalma and Atkinson 2006; Formby 2011b).

Historically, the policy framework has not supported matters of LGBT inclusion. The infamous 'Section 28', for instance, forbade English, Welsh and Scottish local authorities (although ironically not schools) from 'promoting' homosexuality as a 'pretended family relationship' and created a climate of fear regarding teaching about LGB identities or relationships, the legacy of which still remains (Greenland and Nunney 2008). More specifically, the most recent (English) governmental guidance on SRE (DfEE 2000: 4) continues to 'promote' the importance of (by definition, heterosexual) marriage[1] for child-rearing and 'family life'. In addition, personal, social, health and economic education (PSHE) within which some, though not all, of this teaching could fall remains non-statutory in England, resulting in 'patchy' practice (Formby and Wolstenholme 2012). Recent cuts to youth and mental health services in the UK (Puffett 2013a, b) are also likely to impact upon LGBT support in both the statutory and voluntary sectors.

A broad range of institutional practices are relevant to addressing public health inequalities and helping create healthy sustainable places which are supportive of all young people, regardless of their gender and/or sexual identities. UK and international research indicates that where schools are more supportive environments, they can lessen the potential for negative outcomes for LGBT pupils (Espelage et al. 2008; Tippett et al. 2010). Ill-health prevention work therefore has a place in both formal and informal curricula/settings, to prevent negative experiences in adolescence impacting upon educational attainment/inequality and/or on mental health/emotional wellbeing (Rivers 2000; Robinson and Espelage 2011).

Drawing on a social model of health, this chapter critiques the growing (individualist) anti-bullying agenda and argues that it risks minimising understandings of biphobia, homophobia and transphobia. Whilst the term homophobia is rooted in psychology (Adam 1998), and not without its problems, it was nevertheless the word most used by participants to denote prejudice towards LGB (and sometimes trans) individuals/groups. The terms heterosexism and heteronormativity may imply a broader, more sociological analysis, but they are not widely understood or used as commonly as the term homophobia. Homophobia is therefore used throughout this chapter as shorthand for opposition to same-sex relationships and identities that is embedded within social structures and processes. As O'Brien (2008: 497) notes, 'homophobia differs from the common definition of 'phobia' in that the fear is not rooted in individual experience, but rather in culturally learned prejudices'.

The research and its findings

Study methods

The study employed a two-stage methodology: a self-completion survey of young people (online and paper-based), and a follow-up stage of individual interviews and group discussions with young people, youth workers, and secondary school teachers with a responsibility for PSHE and/or LGBT issues. Utilising and extending existing relationships, recruitment was via schools, youth work settings, and other local authority, NHS and voluntary sector contacts. In total, there were 146 survey respondents and 74 participants involved in qualitative methods (see Table 8.1), including nine one-to-one interviews with staff, and eight discussion groups with young people. This approach was taken to gather a range of in-depth perspectives, drawing on the views and experiences of (minority/marginalised) 'lay' groups to identify and explore the issues linking identities and health. This adds to our understanding of current public health concerns, and enables more flexibility, trust-building and participant input than traditional quantitative and/or biomedical approaches allow (see chapter one for further discussion).

TABLE 8.1 Participant details

Participants	Settings			Total
	School	LGBT-specific youth service	Generic youth service	
Staff	4	3	2	9
Young people (aged 11–21 inclusive)	2 groups (= 26 individuals)	2 groups (= 19 individuals)	4 groups (= 20 individuals)	65
Total	**30**	**22**	**22**	**74**

The sample included both staff and young people who identified as LGB and hetero-sexual, though this chapter draws more heavily on data from LGB young people. Most young people were engaged in compulsory schooling, though a minority were in some form of further education or employment, and a small number were not involved in any education, training or employment. The majority of participants were 'white'. Whilst recognising that issues other than/in addition to sexuality (e.g. ethnicity, social class) are also likely to impact upon experiences of homophobia and/or health inequalities (see chapters 1 and 7), an in-depth analysis of these factors was beyond the scope of this study.

All interviews and discussions were digitally recorded and written up. These tran-scripts, and the open text survey data, were analysed thematically. The chapter draws on this qualitative data, using anonymised extracts from participants, with pseudonyms and some demographic information.

Experiences of homophobia and/or bullying

The study identified a range of experiences of homophobia and/or bullying (verbal and physical), most often from those identifying as LGB, but also those with lesbian or gay parents, and those perceived to be 'different' in some way. To a certain extent, LGB participants appeared to expect and/or 'accept' this bullying, because they were aware of their 'different' status:

> There's going to be people out there that are going to be horrible about it, you've just got to learn to deal with it . . . it's something that comes along with the territory . . . it's the society we live in.
>
> *(Matt, male LGBT youth group member aged 16)*

Though there were overt expressions of disapproval of LGB identities among both staff and young people, the issue of (homophobic) language use was complex. Some young people (including LGB) felt that the negative use of the word 'gay' was not homopho-bic, but others were aware of the potential for offence and/or for it to be understood as 'bullying'. Some (LGB) young people did find the term 'gay' used in this way offensive, and said it made them 'more nervous' about 'coming out' about their sexuality, dem-onstrating that intention and perception were not always synonymous when concerning language use.

Other incidences of homophobia/bullying were more clear/explicit, with illustrative examples provided by a number of young people from different schools, including one person having a 'water' bomb of urine thrown at them whilst at school, and another hav-ing acid thrown at them within a science lesson.

Whilst most experiences of homophobia/bullying among LGB participants related to other pupils, there was also evidence of teachers at a range of schools in the region dem-onstrating discriminatory attitudes towards LGB pupils, which could leave them feeling isolated or vulnerable. Young people recalled teachers' comments that were clearly nega-tive and discriminating:

> No wonder you get bullied because you act so gay.
>
> *(Mark, male LGBT youth group member aged 15)*

> If my son or my daughter was ever gay I'd take them into the back of my garden, tie them to the wall and shoot them with a shotgun.
>
> *(Becky, female LGBT youth group member aged 16)*

Consequences for young people

Policies and practices within schools could also be experienced negatively by LGB pupils. Examples include several schools that made (known) lesbian/gay pupils change for physical education (PE) away from other students, making some feel marginalised and excluded, and contributing to their not attending PE and/or school. This clearly has implications for physical health and educational attainment/inequality. In one case a student who complained about this practice was said to be 'causing a fuss', but elsewhere a student had 'co-operated':

> At the end of the day it was partly my decision to do it 'coz I was scared of stuff that would get said or done.
>
> *(Mark)*

Though there are potential repercussions for physical and sexual health too, the impact of bullying and other homophobic experiences was linked by staff to mental health and emotional wellbeing:

> The impact being gay and being out and being bullied has on young people's mental health is colossal . . . The amount of mental health issues in that group that we know about is immense, the ones we don't know about makes me shudder.
>
> *(Male youth worker A, supports LGBT youth group)*

Some felt that these potential impacts were not always understood by other professionals, whether or not they worked directly with young people:

> I get kids who self-harm, who have eating disorders, who run away from home because it's not challenged . . . [but] some other professionals don't see it [as] being a massive deal.
>
> *(Youth worker A)*

Professional responses

As with young people, there were differing professional opinions about the links between language use and homophobia. Some assumed that the use of particular language was intended to be humorous. This was not always an assumption shared by LGB young people who felt bullied. A minority of staff, however, explicitly linked negative language use to bullying, whether or not they thought that was the original intention:

I think for us it is the isolation that people feel when people make comments that makes them feel bullied, and it is a constant problem that yes they [young people] do use the word gay as a putdown.

(Teacher A, female PSHE lead)

Generally, there was a consensus among young people, both LGB and heterosexual, that schools did not respond to homophobic bullying/language as 'seriously' as they did in relation to other forms of prejudice, with racism always the example cited.

Among LGB participants, there tended to be greater disapproval of what they perceived to be schools' lack of action:

People still get away with it in school, it's a bit disgusting really because the school don't really do anything about it.

(Gareth, male LGBT youth group member aged 14)

The prevalence of, and lack of response to, homophobia in schools was acknowledged by some professionals:

It makes me sad that young people don't feel they can report it but I also think that if they are getting it every day at school they just want a quiet life, they just want to come here, somewhere they can just sit and just be safe . . . and just be themselves and I don't think they get that at school or college.

(Youth worker A)

Illustrations of what were felt to be inappropriate or inadequate responses to bullying by professionals/schools were also provided. These included the student (mentioned above) who had the urine-filled 'water' bomb thrown at them but was not allowed home to change, and the student who had acid thrown at them who was told by the teacher they were 'too busy' to discuss it. Often young people felt that bullying was left unaddressed and/or that their complaints were not believed.

A particular response to bullying, in 'supporting' LGB pupils via counselling, was viewed as problematic by some, whether that related to an assumption of 'blame', or its perceived usefulness:

I was kind of like, hang on a minute, 'coz it kind of made me feel like, 'oh is this my fault now, is there something wrong with me?' . . . You've referred me to this person because you think she'll be able to help me, but you didn't bother to check that she was going to be able to help me or not, so you've wasted my time taking me out of lessons.

(Becky)

A number of young people felt that instead of providing counselling referrals, the schools should have challenged the 'perpetrators' of the bullying.

Valued support

Young people more often valued support which they did not equate with an 'at fault' or 'victim' identity. Many young people appreciated the LGBT-specific youth service they were involved with locally, which facilitated access to specialist and/or peer support:

> You're meeting other young people who have been in the same shoes as you . . . and if you need help you can get it, and you can just talk to people and make new friends who are in the same boat.
>
> *(Gemma, female LGBT youth group member aged 18)*

For more than one participant, this service was seen as making the difference between life and death:

> This is gonna sound really dramatic but I'd probably be dead if I never came here . . . because of the amount of bullying that you get and the way that people talk to you, the way that people react . . . you feel like crap, it's either someone's gonna end everything for you, or you're gonna end it for yourself.
>
> *(Becky)*

The safety, confidentiality and identity validation that these environments provided were often said to be crucial because of the fear young people reported related to coming out to parents and/or other staff. Specialist professionals and services were therefore important in supporting wellbeing. However, whilst specialist provision was often viewed as necessary, some staff expressed caution in case it was assumed that young LGBT people automatically need support. This may well be a hard balance to strike: to offer or provide young (LGBT) people support, at the same time as not assuming or implying everyone has a need for it.

Examining professional practices

Where incidences of homophobia were conceptualised as bullying, particularly in relation to language use, this was likely to determine the approach schools might take. Whilst some were more likely to respond to the 'victim' than the 'perpetrator' (e.g. through counselling), others were keen to frame their response within a 'zero tolerance' approach. This meant silencing or stopping all 'inappropriate' language use within an anti-bullying strategy, which met with some teacher support. Some youth workers, however, were more likely to want to give young people the 'permission' to voice potential homophobia, in order to generate discussion, and hopefully, in the long run, greater awareness and/or changed attitudes.

In practice terms, it depended whether voicing particular opinions was interpreted as bullying, and therefore punishable, or whether those opinions were interpreted as a 'right' for those young people, albeit perhaps something to be 'worked on' or 'worked with'. This latter approach arguably requires more complex input and time commitment from staff, and explicitly means giving young people the space to voice potential disapproval of LGB identities and relationships, which may not be compatible with the power dynamics and resources available within schools.

Application to policy and practice

This study broadens existing literature in looking at youth work settings as well as schools, and emphasises the prevalence of homophobia in some young people's lives, which can limit their capabilities, control and ability to prevent ill-health, whether emotional or physical. Drawing on a social model of health, homophobia is a wider problem influencing the settings young people frequent, rather than an individualised problem of bullying. How ever the problem is understood, there is clear potential for negative experiences in adolescence to impact upon emotional health and wellbeing, or a positive sense of self. Those working with young (LGBT) people therefore need to maximise the potential for meeting Marmot review objectives. Possible ways forward from the findings are now discussed.

Capabilities and control

Young LGBT people may need access to 'safe space', specialist expertise and/or peer support. These can be facilitated through LGBT groups supported by a designated worker, but care needs to be taken to not assume that all LGBT young people will want/need this (see Formby 2012 for further discussion of 'safe spaces'). Equally, individual support may be required but care should be taken to not imply any LGBT 'fault' or inherent 'victim' status, and crucially to ensure that the young person wants the support on offer. An alternative/additional way to support LGBT young people is to help them feel that their identities are 'accepted' and 'normal' by facilitating access to affirming events such as Pride,[2] even when this may have to be kept confidential from their parents for safety reasons (Formby 2012 explains the importance of Pride events to LGBT wellbeing).

More broadly, stronger governmental support for appropriate PSHE and/or SRE could facilitate greater LGBT inclusion within schools. This is not to suggest that these are the only curriculum areas where LGBT identities should feature, but that if delivered well and afforded status within schools, these subjects can provide space for young people to explore their own identities and wellbeing, as well as those of others.

Healthy places

If one follows the argument that the problems of homophobia and transphobia exist within wider society, then the solutions to those problems also lie in broader contexts, not just with individuals. This means that concern for young LGBT people's wellbeing should be addressed at a whole-school level, rather than just focusing on known individuals. There needs to be far greater inclusion of LGBT identities within mainstream schooling and youth work practice, rather than a focus on tackling bullying and/or 'supporting' LGBT young people (though this may also need to be provided). Arguments for inclusion can therefore be based more on equalities/diversities and public health agendas than anti-bullying and support needs agendas, which is not to suggest support services should not still be in place. If homophobia is 'culturally learned' (O'Brien 2008) or facilitated, as evidenced in this study, and has implications for health inequalities, schools and youth work settings need to acknowledge the relevance and significance for *all* young people, and staff.

Ill-health prevention

Ideally, future policy and practice would broaden the agenda from bullying to also addressing the potential health implications of heterosexism, homophobia and transphobia, in the first instance by making LGBT identities visible across formal and informal curricula. Sometimes lack of visibility could be addressed as easily as displaying relevant posters (such as advertising local Pride events), or using more inclusive (gender-neutral) language, and not only in PSHE or LGBT-specific youth provision. This may involve support for staff who feel unconfident or unskilled in this area. LGBT history month is a useful resource to demonstrate how LGBT identities have historically been rendered invisible and/or inferior, and how current practice can begin to address this imbalance (see http://lgbthistorymonth.org.uk). The LGB charity Stonewall[3] also offer resources/services which some local authorities (such as Sheffield) engage with via the education champions programme.

A 'joined-up' approach to LGBT public health could see public health professionals looking to examine less common sites of public health practice, such as schools and youth work settings, and could see workers in these same sites engaging more with public health issues. Public health's move from NHS to local authority jurisdiction could encourage this dialogue in the future, if practitioners, and crucially academies and free schools (see Hirst chapter), are willing to engage.

Notes

1 Although as of March 2014 same-sex couples will also be able to legally marry in England and Wales.
2 Pride events celebrate LGBT communities, and often mark the history of the LGBT rights movement. They take place in many locations around the world.
3 See www.stonewall.org.uk.

References

Adam, B. D. (1998) Theorizing homophobia. *Sexualities* 1, 4: 387–404.
Buston, K. (2004) Addressing the sexual health needs of young lesbian, gay and bisexual people. In E. Burtney and M. Duffy (eds) *Young People and Sexual Health: Individual, Social, and Policy Contexts*. Basingstoke: Palgrave Macmillan, pp. 114–127.
DePalma, R. and Atkinson, E. (2006) The sound of silence: talking about sexual orientation and schooling. *Sex Education* 6, 4: 333–349.
DfEE (Department for Education and Employment) (2000) *Sex and Relationship Education Guidance*. Nottingham: DfEE.

Ellis, V. and High, S. (2004) Something more to tell you: gay, lesbian or bisexual young people's experiences of secondary schooling. *British Educational Research Journal* 30, 2: 213–225.

Espelage, D. L., Aragon, S. R., Birkett, M. and Koenig, B. W. (2008) Homophobic teasing, psychological outcomes, and sexual orientation among high school students: what influence do parents and schools have? *School Psychology Review* 37, 2: 202–216.

Fish, J. (2007) *Reducing Health Inequalities for Lesbian, Gay, Bisexual and Trans people.* London: Department of Health.

Formby, E. (2011a) Lesbian and bisexual women's human rights, sexual rights and sexual citizenship: negotiating sexual health in England. *Culture, Health and Sexuality* 13, 10: 1165–1179.

Formby, E. (2011b) Sex and relationships education, sexual health, and lesbian, gay and bisexual sexual cultures: views from young people. *Sex Education* 11, 3: 255–266.

Formby, E. (2012) *Solidarity but not Similarity? LGBT Communities in the Twenty-First Century.* Sheffield: Sheffield Hallam University.

Formby, E. and Wolstenholme, C. (2012) 'If there's going to be a subject that you don't have to do . . .' Findings from a mapping study of PSHE education in English secondary schools, *Pastoral Care in Education* 30, 1: 5–18.

Greenland, K. and Nunney, R. (2008) The repeal of Section 28: it ain't over 'til it's over. *Pastoral Care in Education* 26, 4: 243–251.

King, M., Semlyen, J., See Tai, S., Killaspy, H., Osborn, D., Popelyuk, D. and Nazareth, I. (2008) A systematic review of mental disorder, suicide, and deliberate self harm in lesbian, gay and bisexual people. *BMC Psychiatry* 8, 70.

McNamee, H., Lloyd, K. and Schubotz, D. (2008) Same sex attraction, homophobic bullying and mental health of young people in Northern Ireland. *Journal of Youth Studies* 11, 1: 33–46.

McNeil, J., Bailey, L., Ellis, S., Morton, J. and Regan, M. (2012) *Trans Mental Health Study 2012.* Edinburgh: Scottish Transgender Alliance.

O'Brien, J. (2008) Afterword: Complicating homophobia. *Sexualities* 11, 4: 496–512.

Puffett, N. (2013a) Councils cut back on young people's mental health services. *Children and Young People Now* 11.3.2013.

Puffett, N. (2013b) Councils slash youth services spending by a quarter. *Children and Young People Now* 29.1.2013.

Rivers, I. (2000) Social exclusion, absenteeism and sexual minority youth. *Support for Learning* 15, 1: 13–19.

Rivers, I. and Noret, N. (2008) Well-being among same-sex and opposite-sex attracted youth at school. *School Psychology Review* 37, 2: 174–187.

Robinson, J. P. and Espelage, D. L. (2011) Inequalities in educational and psychological outcomes between LGBTQ and straight students in middle and high school. *Educational Researcher* 40, 7: 315–330.

Tippett, N., Houlston, C. and Smith, P. K. (2010) *Prevention and Response to Identity-Based Bullying among Local Authorities in England, Scotland and Wales.* Manchester: Equality and Human Rights Commission.

Valentine, G., Skelton, T. and Butler, R. (2003) Coming out and outcomes: negotiating lesbian and gay identities with, and in, the family. *Environment and Planning D: Society and Space* 21, 4: 479–499.

Warwick, I., Aggleton, P. and Douglas, N. (2001) Playing it safe: addressing the emotional and physical health of lesbian and gay pupils in the U.K. *Journal of Adolescence* 24, 1: 129–140.

9

EARLY ADULTHOOD (AGES 17–24)

Chris Bentley

Introduction

This part of the life course, as young people develop into adults, is a critical one. It is a time when the potential for positive possibilities regarding health, self-esteem and skills and competencies to protect health can be supported, practised and consolidated. However, it is also the time when harmful behaviours might become established which affect life chances. Many, across the social gradient and due to a plethora of reasons, become involved in practices that can jeopardize their current and future health. Nearly two-thirds of premature deaths and one-third of the total disease burden in adults are associated with conditions or behaviours that began in younger life (WHO 2013). Such behaviours include addiction (e.g. tobacco, alcohol and drugs, lack of physical activity and unprotected sex) and related hazards and health conditions, such as HIV and blood-borne viruses, violence, accident and injury.

Mental health, particularly anxiety or depression, can be a major issue. The risk is increased by experiences of violence, humiliation, isolation, marginalisation, devaluation and poverty, and suicide is one of the leading causes of death in young people (WHO 2013). Building life skills and providing young adults with psychosocial support in schools, colleges and community settings can help promote mental health.

In this section, Chapters 10 and 11 provide two examples of different types of intervention in the Early Adulthood period of the Life Course. These illustrate the potential contribution that qualitative research can make to develop the necessary insight and inform delivery of effective, evidence-based practice that can contribute to ameliorating or preventing negative or unwanted outcomes.

Influencing and supporting behaviour change: breastfeeding

As part of the Life Course approach, the Marmot Report considers Early Adulthood as an important period for intervention not just for the future health and wellbeing of young adults themselves, but also to support giving every child the best start in life (The Marmot Review 2010).

Early adult years can, of course, be a very fertile reproductive period, and parenthood can arise intentionally, and also as an unplanned event. All parents need support at times, and nearly all parents need to turn to someone for information or advice at some point, particularly if they are first time parents, which many in this age group are. Negative situations can be exacerbated where parents are very young, have other challenges in their lives and receive little support from family, peers, health and social care or community.

In particular, when summarising the key interventions through which this age group can contribute to giving every child the best start in life, Marmot recognises two important components (The Marmot Review 2010: 174):

- Priority for maternal health interventions
- Evidence-based parenting support programmes, advice and assistance

Chapter 10 of this book concentrates on an evaluation of an intervention that will potentially impact on both of these components – support for breastfeeding. Breastfeeding has a major role to play in public health, as it promotes health and prevents disease in both the short and long term for both infant and mother.

Breastfeeding initiation rates in the UK have been reported as amongst the lowest in Europe, with rapid discontinuation rates for those who start. Initiation rates and duration rates are lowest for families in the lowest socio-economic groups, adding to inequalities in health and helping to perpetuate the cycle of deprivation. The rates are particularly low among white women in the UK. Teenage or young mothers have also been identified as a vulnerable group, as they are half as likely as older mothers to initiate any breastfeeding (Griffiths et al. 2005).

Programmes that aim to address these characteristics need to consider all potential mechanisms to make a 'sea-change' in population behaviours. A range of such methods were discussed in Chapter 2 of this book, brought together as the 'Population Intervention Triangle'. The different components of the triangle can all potentially make a difference on their own, but will have the greatest chance of significant impact if all are deployed in a cohesive strategy delivered across a committed partnership.

Components of a strategy to achieve a percentage change improvement in breastfeeding initiation and continuation at population level will apply and have relevance, proportionately across the social gradient. However, there are some parts of society that will still need 'disproportionate' inputs if they are to achieve even average outcomes. In relation to breastfeeding one such grouping consists of teenagers and young mothers and those influencing decision-making, such as fathers and wider family members.

A specific evidence-based action that is recommended is the development of local media programmes targeting teenagers to improve and shift attitudes towards breastfeeding (NICE 2006). It is stated that the media has a strong influence on young girls. However, each media campaign should be developed locally, using locally produced images, in relation to specific target groups. The content should be based on user experiences and viewpoints, and not those of health professionals.

In Chapter 10 Lindsay Reece and Anna Clack use a qualitative evaluation of one such programme to examine the strengths and weaknesses of the process.

Strengthening the role of ill-health prevention: drawing young adults into services

The Marmot Report makes a call to: 'Prioritise prevention and early detection of those conditions most strongly related to health inequalities' (The Marmot Review 2010: 190). There is a linked policy recommendation to 'Implement evidence-based programmes of ill-health preventive interventions that are effective across the social gradient'.

Emphasis is placed on the evidence-based interventions in the NICE (National Institute of Health and Clinical Excellence) programme, and therefore, the intention is greater use of cost-effective preventive interventions. This should, in due course, deliver a reduction in preventable and avoidable death and disability. Many NICE systematic reviews find differential impacts of health inequalities on interventions, but are often 'light' in equity impact assessment, as there is little supporting evidence to be found that meets their criteria. These criteria, may however, exclude forms of evidence as described in the Leeds Declaration, as providing invaluable information to help develop useful public health programmes.

The 'Decay model' of the fall-off in uptake of evidence-based protocol interventions, such as those specified by NICE, was presented in Chapter 2 of this book. This has shown that there is a tendency for only a small percentage of people who could possibly benefit to actually achieve the desirable results of the treatment or therapy.

The case study described by Ray Poll in Chapter 11 is an example of how good qualitative research can provide important insight at a number of important points A–D in the model, in support of NICE guidelines (NICE 2012). The group he has accessed, people with a history of intravenous drug use and risk of hepatitis C, can be marginalised, assumed to have chaotic lives, and therefore being 'poor' users of conventional services. However, it could also be the case that the services are not best adapted to the needs of their particular client group. The consequences of not accessing services that can screen and either treat or help prevent infection, can be catastrophic. The infection itself can be acutely unpleasant, and can lead to severe and fatal liver disease. If infection is not controlled and managed, there can be an expanding reservoir of infection, with important public health consequences.

The study provides important points of insight, and is able to recommend practical actions providing the real possibility of improvement in the services offered.

References

Griffiths, L. J., Dezateux, C. and Law, C. (2005) The contribution of parental and community ethnicity to breastfeeding practices: evidence from the Millennium Cohort Study. *International Journal of Epidemiology* 34: 1378–1386.

Marmot Review (2010) *Fair Society, Healthy Lives*. London: The Marmot Review.

NICE (2006) *Promotion of Breastfeeding Initiation and Duration: Evidence into Practice Briefing*. London: National Institute for Health and Care Excellence.

NICE (2012) *Hepatitis B and C: Ways to Promote and Offer Testing to People at Increased Risk of Infection. NICE Public Health Guidance* 43. London: NICE.

WHO (2013) *Young People: Health Risks and Solutions*. Fact sheet 345. Geneva: WHO.

10

BREASTFEEDING

Engaging teenage mothers in healthy lifestyle change

Lindsey Reece and Anna Clack

Introduction

The health and wellbeing of all women before, during and after pregnancy is a critical factor in giving children the best start in life (Marmot 2010). The health of babies is critically affected by the health and wellbeing of mothers (Marmot 2010). In areas of high deprivation, the health of babies and some young mothers is poorer than those in more affluent areas. At national level it is recognised that supporting young people to be healthy is a valuable investment in the country's future (Department of Health 2008). The Social Exclusion Unit (1999) report, which has laid the foundations of government policy since that time, stated teenage pregnancy was a major social and economic problem. The United Kingdom ranked unfavourably when compared to other Westernised nations. Duncan, Edwards and Alexander (2010) questioned this, citing evidence that pregnancy, at any age could be seen as an opportunity to establish the foundations of healthy lifestyle practices for mothers, their babies and their families (Foresight 2007; NICE 2011, 2010).

Breastfeeding is a global health priority. The World Health Organisation (WHO) recommends exclusive breastfeeding for six months, followed by the appropriate introduction of solids, and continued breastfeeding for two years and beyond (World Health Organisation 2003). This recommendation is supported by robust evidence detailing the short and long term health benefits for both mother and infant (McInnes et al. 2013), particularly in low-income countries where its relevance for child survival is undisputed (UNICEF 2011).

Globally, breastfeeding rates are low. Rates in some regions including Europe are steadily rising, for example in France, Italy, the Netherlands, Spain and Switzerland. Sweden leads the way with a prevalence of 98 per cent (WHO Global Data Bank 2013). In the UK, non-adherence to the WHO recommendations is typical with only 1 per cent of babies exclusively breastfed in 2010 (Health and Social Care Information Centre 2012). Initial breastfeeding rates (including all babies who were put to the breast at all) were 81 per cent in 2010, yet the steepest drop-off in breastfeeding occurs in the first few weeks of life, reinforcing the need for effective interventions to support mothers to maintain breastfeeding for longer. As it stands, effectiveness of these targets and interventions is limited (Bartington et al. 2006).

In all countries (including the UK), at all levels of income, health and illness, breastfeeding rates follow a social gradient: the lower the socio-economic position the worse the health outcomes (Health and Social Care Information Centre 2012; Marmot 2010). A significant proportion of new born babies are therefore not receiving the optimal nutritional start in life (Bartington et al. 2006). The importance of breastfeeding-related health outcomes in reducing health inequalities has been firmly acknowledged in the UK, leading to an increased drive to increase initiation rates among those living with high deprivation and young mothers as an identified priority group (Department of Health 2004).

This chapter focuses on a study which contributes to understanding young women's breastfeeding decisions and behaviour in contexts of living in deprived communities. It explores their decisions regarding healthy lifestyles and their interaction with the healthcare system. The data evolved from evaluating the impact of a teenage breastfeeding campaign, in Rotherham, South Yorkshire. The evaluation was a small qualitative study involving interviews and focus groups (Braun and Clarke 2006). The context, findings and implications for policy and practice are summarised in this chapter.

Underpinning theory and policy

Despite levels of teenage conception being at a 20-year low, rates in the UK are amongst the highest in Western Europe (Viner and Booy 2005). The reasons for teenage conceptions and parenthood remain contested and are complex. Agreement exists on the most significant determinants (Duncan et al. 2010), with a consensus that young adults who continue a pregnancy are primarily from socio-economically deprived backgrounds (UNICEF 2012) and experience higher rates of infant mortality compared to more affluent population groups. Marmot (2010) pointed to infant mortality as the leading indicator of health inequality.

In the UK, generally, teenage mothers are less likely to finish their education, more likely to be unemployed (Social Exclusion Unit 1999), experience poor mental health, have lower predicted child health outcomes, experience ante-natal health concerns (UNICEF 2012) and are less likely to engage with healthcare services, all of which perpetuates the cycle of deprivation (Arthur et al. 2007). In contrast to this, some teenage mothers, and their children, live happy and fulfilling lives (Duncan et al. 2010). Research indicates that some of the adversities associated with teen parenthood have been exaggerated, with poverty being more significant than the age of first motherhood (Ermisch and Pevalin 2003). Duncan et al. (2007) propose that teenage pregnancy is rarely a catastrophe and that teenage parenting does not specifically cause poor health outcomes for mother and baby: it can, in fact be a positive experience, a turning point, for young mothers and fathers.

Undoubtedly, pregnancy presents a critical point in a women's life, irrespective of age, for a change to occur. Whilst a 'whole-systems' approach to tackling health inequalities is required (Marmot 2010), interventions that support young mothers to adopt healthy lifestyles, enhance their capability to self-manage long-term conditions and encourage them to initiate and maintain breastfeeding (Department of Health 2004, 2012) are all likely to make a significant contribution to ensuring children have the best start in life and build the family's capability to lead a healthier lifestyle. Providing an alternative socio-economic trajectory for teenage mothers, one which supports young women to take ownership over their health and the future health of their baby, must remain a priority for public health intervention, as outlined by Marmot (2010).

In light of these challenges for mothers aged 19 and under it is important to better understand how best to engage young women with support services early on in their pregnancy journey. In this way appropriate services can be delivered that encourage them to adopt healthy lifestyles for themselves and for their child postnatally. One such strategy is the promotion of breastfeeding; the remainder of this chapter focuses on one such initiative.

Breast is best?

The importance of breastfeeding-related health outcomes in reducing health inequalities has been firmly acknowledged in the UK, with investment in campaigns such as UNICEF Baby Friendly (UNICEF 2011) to support women to breastfeed. Young women living in deprived communities tend to follow their family pattern which reinforces low breastfeeding rates. As has been repeatedly recommended, the promotion of breastfeeding and the development of campaigns to aid women to breastfeed are among the most effective early years strategies to tackle health inequalities and improve general health (Field 2010; Marmot 2010). Despite this, a recent survey found that effective care for breastfeeding is often insufficient (Health and Social Care Information Centre 2012). Systematic reviews also indicate inconsistent effectiveness of intervention with outcomes varying according to socio-economic status (Renfrew et al. 2012). Further exploration is required into the most appropriate way to engage young women, and break reproduction of social norms.

Benefits of breastfeeding

The wider benefits of breastfeeding for mother as well as infant health are well documented (Department of Health 2004; WHO 2003). These include reducing weight gained during pregnancy, reducing the potential risk of obesity for their children in later life, and providing improved immune function and protection against allergies (Armstrong and Reilly 2002).

The optimal length of time to breastfeed is debated, yet the WHO recommendation currently remains best practice (WHO 2003). Initiation rates have steadily increased over the years (Health and Social Care 2012) yet no significant increase has been seen amongst teenage mothers. Maintenance rates at six weeks are also yet to see an increase by the same margin for mothers irrespective of age. It is hypothesised that this initiation increase is due to the increased public and professional awareness of the impact of infant feeding on health (Department of Health 2007; NICE 2011; UNICEF 2011). However, further work is needed to encourage and support young, teenage, women to continue breastfeeding for longer. Several reasons for the early cessation of breastfeeding in the UK include perception of pain, physical pain of breastfeeding, newborn struggling to thrive and mother returning to work (Dyson et al. 2006). There is an acceptance amongst communities that formula feeding is a 'normal' and safe way to feed babies and this therefore generates an unsympathetic attitude towards breastfeeding (Dyson et al. 2010) creating an additional barrier for young women to choose to breastfeed.

In summary, breastfeeding rates in the UK remain low across all age groups but younger mothers from socially disadvantaged communities are less likely to initiate breastfeeding, and if they do so are more likely to stop breastfeeding earlier (Griffiths et al. 2009; Scott and Mostyn 2003). Only 52 per cent women under the age of 20 years old initiate breastfeeding at birth, with only 32 per cent of those still breastfeeding at one week (Bolling et al. 2007).

The Baby Friendly Hospital Initiative (BFHI) is one of many policies aimed at increasing breastfeeding across the UK (UNICEF 2011). In accordance with the Global Strategy on Infant and Young Child Feeding (WHO 2003), UNICEF's overall goal is to protect, promote and support optimal infant and young child feeding practices. In the UK, *Maternity Matters* guidance (Department of Health 2007) specified the requirement for high quality, safe and accessible maternity services that were family focused as well as concentrating on the more vulnerable and disadvantaged families. This reflects Marmot's primary objective (Marmot 2010).

In the light of existing research and policy, there appears an argument for further development of teenage-specific maternity care services. In an attempt to overcome the barriers faced by young women living in deprived communities, a national campaign in the UK, 'Be a Star', was developed as one of the first social marketing campaigns specifically targeting breastfeeding in young women. This chapter now reflects on selected findings of an evaluation of 'Be a Star'.

The research and its findings

England average breastfeeding initiation rates were 74 per cent, with breastfeeding continuation rates at 6–8 weeks 47.2 per cent in 2011/12 (ChiMat 2013). Historically, Rotherham has lower rates than the England average with initiation rates of 61.5 per cent with 31.2 per cent continuing until 6–8 weeks point (Child and Maternal Health 2013). Even more worrying, however, are the continuous low rates amongst the teenage group; as a result increasing breastfeeding initiation and maintenance rates amongst young adults became a public health priority. The 'Be a Star' breastfeeding campaign was launched in Rotherham, targeting women aged 18–25 years from areas of high deprivation across the city. The campaign aimed to increase the number of young mothers choosing to breastfeed by showcasing local young mothers, photographed in poses of their choosing, feeding their babies whilst detailing the benefits of breastfeeding and offering practical tips on how to breastfeed (Rotherham NHS Foundation Hospital Trust 2012) (see Figure 10.1). The campaign showcases local women and the pride, sense of beauty and confidence

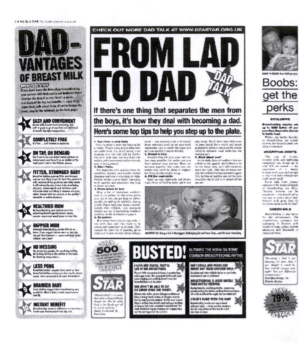
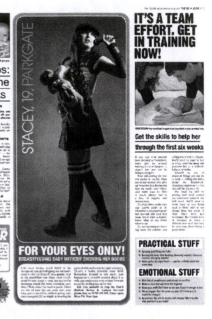
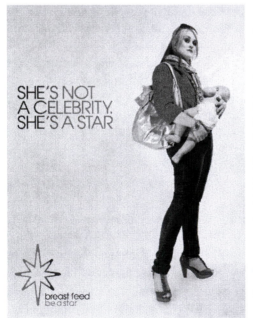
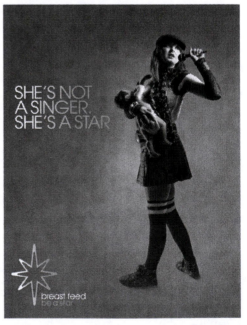

FIGURE 10.1 Images from the 'Be a Star' breastfeeding campaign (http://www. collaborativechange.org.uk. © Collaborative Change 2013. Reproduced with permission).

that can be achieved by breastfeeding. It focuses on supporting women to feel a sense of achievement and satisfaction for breastfeeding and providing their baby with the best start in life, as well as providing hints and tips on breastfeeding in public. The campaign has a broad portfolio of educational resources (billboards; leaflets; internet and social media sites; a dad's magazine).

Methods

A study was conducted to explore breastfeeding experiences and evaluate awareness of the 'Be a star' campaign amongst young women aged between 15 and 25 years old living in deprived communities. Young women were recruited through community peer support groups, hospital and community maternity services. A mixture of telephone interviews (n = 9) and focus groups (n = 21) were conducted. A thematic analysis (Braun and Clarke 2006) was conducted by three independent researchers, in order to identify, analyse and report key emerging themes.

Research findings

The breastfeeding decision

Overall, the evaluation revealed a positive attitude towards breastfeeding amongst the participants. The breastfeeding decision, for many, was not thought through, with very few young women remembering a specific time point at which a decision was made; it was the 'right thing to do' (Mum 2). There was a definite 'give it a go' (Mum 3) mentality driven by their personal values.

> There is that fighting spirit inside that says [. . .] I'm not going to be beaten by this, I can do it.
>
> *(Mum 4)*

Moreover, some young women were influenced by a positive interaction with healthcare services. This implies that a positive experience with the healthcare system early on in the maternal care pathway can encourage future engagement with health services, which is a priority amongst this young population (Arthur et al. 2007).

> I just wanted to breastfeed from the day I found out I was pregnant, just because it's best for her.
>
> *(Mum 5)*

The decision to breastfeed was further influenced by social norms; the surrounding environment and relationships with family and friends. Young girls were more likely to breastfeed if they had friends and relatives who had breastfed, if they had seen others feeding and/or were breastfed themselves.

The primary barrier to breastfeeding that emerged related to socio-cultural influences, and the perception that bottle feeding is the norm. Young participants reported seeing bottle feeding more often on television and portrayed as less problematic (Scott and Mostyn 2003). Breastfeeding in public is not commonplace in the UK, and social expectations require breastfeeding to be conducted in a discreet way (Bolling et al. 2007). Participants who had attempted to breastfeed in public spoke of a perceived stigma which negatively impacted on their confidence and self-esteem. This is echoed in the three-generation study of teenage parenting by Hirst et al. (2006) and by Bolling et al. (2007) who reported over 40 per cent of women had received negative reactions of some kind from members of the public when breastfeeding in public places.

> The more and more you see it the less you're going to get stared at because you're not singling yourself out by sitting and getting your boob out and feeding your baby, which obviously is natural, but not everybody sees it like that.
>
> *(Mum 6)*

Breast is best

The findings indicate that the positive impact of breastfeeding on the health and that of their babies was a main motivation to initiate breastfeeding.

> wanted to give it a go, even if couldn't do it for long, try for my baby's sake!
>
> *(Mum 7)*

This strong consensus amongst participants that 'breast is best' implies that knowledge of the benefits of breastfeeding was not a limiting factor in the decision to breastfeed yet did not help encourage them to sustain breastfeeding their baby.

> Something the literature doesn't say, whilst it's the most natural thing in the world [breastfeeding], it's not the easiest thing to do . . . and it hurts like hell!
>
> *(Mum 5)*

Many of these women found the experience much more difficult than they had expected. This is in line with previous findings, suggesting that early cessation of breastfeeding relates to women's perceived difficulty with breastfeeding (Dykes et al. 2003). Other reasons for stopping breastfeeding included sore nipples, technical issues such as latching on, and inability to satisfy babies' needs. This emphasises the requirement for practical and skilled support. Emotionally, young women found the experience stressful and demanding, with these feelings increasing, and self-confidence diminishing, the longer it went on.

Service provision and support

A quantifiable positive effect of breastfeeding is the increase in a mother's self-esteem and confidence if she successfully initiates breastfeeding, and this was particularly notable in our study. Young women spoke of feeling proud, wanting to be a role model for their child and having their self-worth reinforced. This can be fostered through the provision of client-centred, non-judgemental, empathetic pregnancy services, which offer young women positive reinforcement and feedback on their progress.

I remember having those odd days . . . thinking I don't want to do this anymore, and just knowing that there's someone there that can say it's not going to be like this forever.

(Mum 2)

I know this will hurt but you know what, you can do this, come on you are doing great!

(Mum 8)

A desire to receive pragmatic, honest and realistic advice, at the right time, from health professionals was expressed by the participants in this research. The discrepancy between the perceived difficulty of breastfeeding and the actual experience was marked, and in the majority of cases this leads to early cessation.

Literature's all right if it's given at the point you need it. You seem to get bombarded at the beginning with lots, and then as stages go by that you need it you don't know where to look for it.

(Mum 9)

Application to practice

A fundamental question emerging from this study relates to the content, frequency and timing of support provided throughout the maternal care pathway. Participants' experiences indicate ante–natal focus should be on the benefits of breastfeeding and setting the scene for what lies ahead. For many participants the decision was innate and dependent upon previous experience and their environment and upbringing. Ante-natal care can optimise engagement with the health service, and establish or strengthen existing support networks ready for when the baby is born by delivering client-centred support. This enhances an individual's confidence and self-esteem so that young mothers have greater potential to breastfeed and overcome barriers that they might face. This reinforces the need for further exploration into the appropriate content, timing and intensity of support delivered to young women (Giles et al. 2010).

Post-natal advice delivered by health services could focus on practical and technical advice positively reinforcing progress in a friendly approachable manner. This not only has the potential to influence breastfeeding rates but also could help reduce the perceived stigma felt by young women in response to their engagement with healthcare professionals.

There is a strong preference amongst young women in this study to receive open, honest and realistic advice in post-natal care about the breastfeeding experience. This could focus on positive encouragement, practical and technical advice, alongside friendly, skilled support to help sustain breastfeeding for a longer period.

Many of the young mothers who took part in this study have a strong, resilient sense of identity. They have grit and determination to become good parents, overcome adversity and provide their child with the best start in life. This assertion is backed up by numerous studies (see Duncan et al. 2010, for overview).

Previous information campaigns have focused on initiation and the benefits of breast-feeding yet this research suggests knowledge is not the issue. Positive reinforcement, confidence building, and pragmatic and realistic service delivery by healthcare professionals designed with the needs of young women in mind should be the priority.

The decision to breastfeed is arguably not a conscious one; it is influenced by social norms, environment and relationships with family and friends. This highlights the importance of fostering a breastfeeding friendly culture and encouraging young people to be role models for future generations.

Consideration could also be given to exploring the appropriate frequency, intensity and timing of support. Sarafino (1994) outlines five main components of support. The current focus of breastfeeding support for young women is driven by information-giving advice and network support through the establishment of peer support groups. There is an apparent gap in support that relates to the emotional and self-esteem aspects of breast-feeding in young women, which shifts the focus to expressing empathy and positively reinforcing individuals' aspirations, ideas and feelings. This was outlined when considering support needed to increase duration of breastfeeding. The focus must be on emotional, esteem and instrumental support (Sarafino 1994). A benefit of conducting focus groups and interviews with young women in this study was that the views of the women themselves could be explored, giving them a voice which may not have been heard in other forums.

Conclusion

This chapter has considered the health inequality landscape surrounding young women in deprived communities. The chapter provides insight into existing health inequalities that prevent children in some communities having the best start in life. It highlights important aspects and influences surrounding breastfeeding experiences, breastfeeding beliefs and breastfeeding initiation and maintenance in young women living in deprived communities. Findings can be used to develop public health practice.

Many of the young women in this evaluation had negative experiences related to breastfeeding, yet their resilience, in overcoming the barriers and giving breastfeeding a go, was evident. As Marmot (2010) outlines, this must be fostered to enable all young people to maximise their capabilities to take control over their lives. This will then help give all children the best start in life and contribute to preventing ill health among mothers and their children.

References

Armstrong, J. and Reilly, J. (2002) Breastfeeding and lowering the risk of childhood obesity. *Lancet* 359: 2003–2004.

Arthur, A., Unwin, S. and Mitchell, T. (2007) Teenage mothers' experiences of maternity services: a qualitative study. *British Journal of Midwifery* 15, 11: 672–677.

Bartington, S., Griffiths, L., Tate, L. and Dezateux, C. (2006) Are breastfeeding rates higher among mothers delivering in baby friendly accredited maternity units in the UK? *International Journal of Epidemiology* 35, 5: 1178–1186.

Bolling, K., Grant, C., Hamlyn, B. and Thornton, A. (2007) *Infant Feeding Survey 2005*. London: The Information Centre for Health and Social Care and the UK Health Departments.

Braun, V. and Clarke, B. (2006) Using thematic analysis in psychology. *Qualitative Research in Psychology* 3, 2: 77–101.

Child and Maternal Health Intelligence Network (2013) *Breastfeeding Profiles*. Online at: http://www.chimat.org.uk/default.aspx?QN=CHIMAT_DATADIR_MI Accessed September 2013.

Department of Health (2004) *Good Practice and Innovation in Breastfeeding*. London: Department of Health.

Department of Health (2007) *Maternity Matters: Choice, Access and Continuity of Care in a Safe Service*. London: Department of Health.

Department of Health (2008) *2007 Annual Report of the Chief Medical Officer. Tackling the health of the teenage nation*. Online at: http://webarchive.nationalarchives.gov.uk/20130107105354/http://www.dh.gov.uk/prod_consum_dh/groups/dh_digitalassets/@dh/@en/documents/digitalasset/dh_086193.pdf Accessed December 2013.

Department of Health (2012) *Improving Outcomes and Supporting Transparency: Part 1: A Public Health Outcomes Framework for England, 2013–2016*. London: Department of Health.

Duncan, S. (2007) What's the problem with teenage parents? And what's the problem with policy? *Critical Social Policy* 27: 307–334.

Duncan, S., Edwards, R. and Alexander, C. (2010) *Teenage Parenthood: What's the Problem?* London: Tuffnell Press.

Dykes, F., Moran, V., Burt, S. and Edwards, J. (2003) Adolescent mothers and breastfeeding experiences and support needs. *Journal of Human Lactation* 19: 391–401.

Dyson, L., Renfrew, M., McFadden, A., McCormick, F., Herbert, G. and Thomas, J. (2006) *Promoting Breastfeeding Initiation and Duration: Evidence into Practice Briefing*. London: National Institute for Health and Clinical Excellence.

Dyson, L., Green, J., Renfrew, M., McMillan, B. and Woolridge, M. (2010) Factors influencing the infant feeding decision for socioeconomically deprived pregnant teenagers: the moral dimension. Issues in perinatal care. *Birth* 37, 2: 141–149.

Ermisch, J. and Pevalin, D. (2003) *Does a 'Teen-Birth' Have Longer-Term Impacts on the Mother? Evidence from the 1970 British Cohort Study*. ISER Working paper, University of Essex. Online at: https://www.iser.essex.ac.uk/files/iser_working_papers/2003-32.pdf Accessed September 2013.

Field, F. (2010) *The Foundation Years: Preventing Poor Children Becoming Poor Adults. The Report of the Independent Review of Poverty and Life Chances*. London: Cabinet Office.

Foresight (2007) *Tackling Obesity: Future Choices*. Government Office for Science. London: HMSO.

Giles, M., Connor, S., McClenahan, C. and Mallet, J. (2010) Attitudes to breastfeeding among adolescents. *Journal of Human Nutrition and Dietetics* 23: 285–293.

Griffiths, L. J., Smeeth, L., Sherburne Hawkins, S., Cole, T. and Dezateux, C. (2009) Effect of infant feeding practice on weight gain from birth to 3 years. *Archives of Disease in Childhood* 94: 577–582.

Health and Social Care Information Centre (2012) *Infant Feeding Survey 2010* (1st ed.). The NHS Health and Social Care Information Centre. Updated 2012. Online at: http://www.hscic.gov.uk/catalogue/PUB08694 Accessed September 2013.

Hirst, J., Formby, E. and Owen, J. (2006). *Pathways into Parenthood: Reflections from Three Generations of Teenage Mothers and Fathers. Project Report*. Sheffield: Sheffield Hallam University.

McInnes, R., Hoddinott, P., Britten, J., Darwent, K. and Craig, L. (2013) Significant others, situations and infant feeding behaviour change processes: a serial qualitative interview study. *BMC Pregnancy and Childbirth* 13: 114.

Marmot Review (2010) *Fair Society, Healthy Lives*. London: The Marmot Review.

National Institute for Health and Clinical Excellence (2011) *Dietary Interventions and Physical Activity Interventions for Weight Management before, during and after Pregnancy*. London: NICE.

Renfrew, M., McCormick, F., Wade, A., Quinn, B. and Dowswell, T. (2012) *Support for Healthy Breastfeeding Mothers with Healthy Term Babies*. The Cochrane Library. John Wiley. Online at: http://onlinelibrary.wiley.com/doi/10.1002/14651858.CD001141.pub4/pdf/ Accessed September 2013.

Rotherham NHS Foundation Hospital Trust (2012) *Quality Account 2012–2013*. Online at: http://www.nhs.uk/Services/UserControls/UploadHandlers/MediaServerHandler.ashx?id=410 Accessed September 2013.

Sarafino E. P. (1994) *Health Psychology: Biopsychology Interactions*. New York: John Wiley.

Scott, J. and Mostyn, T. (2003) Women's experiences of breastfeeding in a formula feeding culture. *Journal of Human Lactation* 19: 270–277.

Social Exclusion Unit (1999) *Teenage Pregnancy: Report by the Social Exclusion Unit*. London: Stationery Office.

UNICEF (2011) *The Baby Friendly Hospital Initiative*. Online at: http://www.unicef.org.uk/BabyFriendly/About-Baby-Friendly Accessed September 2013.

UNICEF (2012) *Preventing Disease and Saving Resources: The Potential Contribution of Increasing Breastfeeding Rates in the UK*. Online at: http://www.unicef.org.uk/Documents/Baby_Friendly/Research/Preventing_disease_saving_resources.pdf Accessed September 2013.

Viner, R. and Booy, R. (2005) Epidemiology of health and illness: ABC of adolescence. *British Medical Journal* 330 (7488): 411–414.

World Health Organisation (2003) *Global Strategy for Infant and Young Child Feeding*. Geneva: WHO. Online at: http://www.who.int/nutrition/publications/gs_infant_feeding_text_eng.pdf Accessed September 2013.

World Health Organisation (2013) *Global Data Bank on Infant and Young Child Feeding*. Online at: http://www.who.int/nutrition/databases/infantfeeding/en/ Accessed September 2013.

11

PREVENTING ILL-HEALTH

Assessing the potential impact of NICE guidance to promote and offer hepatitis C testing within drug services

Ray Poll

Introduction

Hepatitis C is a blood-borne virus that primarily affects the liver. Without treatment it can cause advanced liver disease (cirrhosis), liver cancer (hepatocellular carcinoma [HCC]) and sometimes death (National Institute for Health and Clinical Excellence [NICE] 2006). Infection disproportionately affects people from the poorest sections of society, who '. . . have not succeeded in education, have little work experience, lack supportive relationships and often suffer with poor mental health . . .' (National Treatment Agency [NTA] 2012: 4). Thus, the lifestyle of those susceptible to infection is embedded in the wider social, environmental and economic determinants of health (Dahlgren and Whitehead 2007). Although hepatitis C is a global health problem, the focus of this chapter is on the UK.

Marmot (2010) proposes that an investment in ill-health prevention will reduce health inequalities, and will improve the health and life expectancy of the population. In this endeavour he recommends using NICE programmes to deliver interventions because they are evidence-based, include an 'inequalities filter' and are assessed for cost-effectiveness (Marmot 2010).

NICE produces evidence-based guidance on treatment, procedures and devices which represent high quality care and value for money for the NHS (NICE 2012a). NICE also produces public health guidance recommending the best ways to prevent disease and promote wellbeing.

This chapter presents some findings from a qualitative research project that explored the reasons for missed appointments at drug service hepatitis C outreach clinics. The findings are used to explore the potential effectiveness of a new piece of NICE guidance (2012b) for promoting and offering testing to people at high risk of hepatitis C (and B). The guidance is in keeping with a priority for Marmot (2010), namely to prevent and diagnose conditions early that are strongly related to health inequalities.

Thus, the chapter comprises three sections:

- The health burden of hepatitis C and current policy to tackle this
- An outline of the research project and some of the findings
- Discussion of the findings and how these might impact on implementation of the testing guidance for hepatitis C.

Theory and policy

The health burden of hepatitis C

There are approximately 123 million people chronically infected with hepatitis C worldwide (Shepard et al. 2005). In England (a low prevalence country), 85,565 people were diagnosed up to 2010, although it is estimated that 161,320 people are actually infected (Health Protection Agency [HPA] 2011). Many people remain undiagnosed, largely because of the asymptomatic nature of infection. About 90 per cent of infections are attributable to injecting drug use, with approximately half from this group infected (HPA 2012a).

Despite the chance of a cure for the majority of chronically infected people, only about 20 per cent were treated between 2006 and 2011, with just 3 per cent treated each year (HPA 2012b). In England it is predicted that, by 2020, approximately 16,000 individuals will be living with cirrhosis or HCC if their hepatitis C remains untreated (HPA 2012b). Not only is there a health burden for people with hepatitis C, but also an escalating cost to health services. Both the number of hospital admissions and liver transplants performed has risen as a result of hepatitis C-related disease (HPA 2012b).

In England (and elsewhere), action plans and work programmes are in place to tackle hepatitis C, with four key areas identified:

(a) The prevention of new infections
(b) Raising awareness of infection
(c) Increasing testing and diagnosis
(d) Engaging infected individuals into care and treatment.

(a) Prevention of new infections

To reduce drug dependence and stop people injecting, opiate substitution therapy, (OST) e.g. methadone, is offered by specialist clinics and some general practitioners (GPs) (NICE 2007). For those who continue to inject, needle and syringe programmes (NSPs) based in drug services and chemists provide clean equipment (NICE 2009). It is argued that a combination of OST, NSPs and the treatment of injecting drug users (IDUs) with hepatitis C may reduce the incidence and prevalence of the infection (Martin et al. 2011).

Marmot (2010) agrees that OST is an essential part of drug policy but reminds services of the need to address peoples' 'individual factors' or social issues e.g. homelessness, to ensure treatment is accessible. He adds that 'medicalising' drug use (*versus* criminalising it), by referring people to drug courts comprising health and social care professionals, can lead to an increased uptake of drug treatment and a reduction in mortality (Marmot

2010), thereby recognising and being inclusive of the wider determinants of health which can negatively impact on access to healthcare services (Dahlgren and Whitehead 2007).

(b) Raising awareness of infection

Reducing undiagnosed infection is a priority, with articles in professional journals, magazines and newspapers and in television and radio programme broadcasts. Internet websites have flourished, including one inviting people to undertake a quick anonymised questionnaire to assess their infection risk (NHS Choices 2012). Leaflets and posters are displayed in general practice surgeries and clinics, and educational sessions are provided for professionals and risk groups in a variety of settings, including hostels and prisons. Recent developments include the Royal College of General Practitioners certificate in hepatitis C (and B) for primary care professionals, and the establishment of World Hepatitis Day (28 July) with testing often available at events.

With a good start in life being fundamental to the avoidance of later inequalities, Marmot (2010) recommends that school children are equipped with knowledge and skills to resist experimenting with drugs and entering a life of addiction.

(c) Increasing testing and diagnosis

To improve access to testing for marginalised groups (including IDUs), this may take place in general practice surgeries, ante-natal clinics, drug misuse services, prisons, and Genito-Urinary Medicine sexual health clinics (Department of Health [DoH], 2004). Locally, two drug service hepatitis C outreach clinics have been established to increase rates of diagnoses (and attendance for treatment) but many patients do not keep their appointment.

New NICE guidance (2012b) to promote and encourage people at risk of infection to be tested has been published. The recommendations for drug services include:

- Identifying a hepatitis lead with knowledge and skills to promote testing and treatment, with consideration given to training peer mentors and health champions to support this work;
- Ensuring that there is a local care pathway into specialist care for infected people, including the possibility of providing treatment in the community combined with OST, and facilitated by access to specialist phlebotomy services;
- Offering and promoting testing to all service users, with annual screening for people who test negative for hepatitis C but remain at risk of infection; and
- Ensuring that staff have the knowledge and skills to promote testing and treatment, and are trained and competent to undertake pre- and post-test discussions and dried blood-spot (DBS) testing (for people with poor venous access).

(d) Engaging infected individuals into care and treatment

Individuals with chronic hepatitis C should be referred for specialist care and treatment (DoH 2002). Hospital-based specialist nurses run clinics to assess patients, and to commence them on treatment and monitor the side-effects of this. However, many people do not engage with health services and remain untreated (Maghlaoui 2012). Non-attendance with the local drug service hepatitis C outreach clinics also means patients miss the opportunity of referral (by this route) to the hospital for care and treatment.

One successful strategy has been to make services more accessible, with treatment provided in non-traditional settings such as prisons, drug misuse services and health centres (Lewis et al. 2012). This provision has been somewhat limited, with expansion recommended (HPA 2012b).

In summary, despite policy and action plans to prevent transmission, to raise awareness and to increase testing, with established pathways into curative treatment, many people with hepatitis C remain undiagnosed or untreated.

There are several possible reasons why people remain untreated: too few specialist nurses to deliver the service; different clinical interpretations of guidelines, with groups of patients treated in some areas and not others; and patients missing appointments (Stephens 2012). The latter is the focus of the qualitative research discussed in this chapter.

Research and findings

This study investigated the reason for missed appointments with drug service hepatitis C outreach clinics. The rationale for the research approach and some of the study findings now follows.

The research approach

In the absence of previous research, the reasons why people with hepatitis C miss clinic appointments appear uncertain. Explanations are often based on assumptions of 'chaotic lifestyles' and that people are 'hard-to-reach'. It could be argued that these terms blame individuals for their ill-health and non-engagement with health services, and fail to examine 'upstream' wider social and economic determinants of health (Dahlgren and Whitehead 2007). The Leeds Declaration in 1993 suggested that public health's past reliance on traditional epidemiological data from bio-medical quantitative studies must be challenged, with gaps in understanding filled by using more appropriate qualitative methods (Long 1994). As well as making sense of the causes of ill-health, lay people's knowledge is important in understanding their experience of health services. They are likely to ascribe different experiences and meanings to health and illness that are not always captured using quantitative methods.

Having identified a gap in knowledge this study sought explanations from patients about missing appointments. Qualitative semi-structured interviews enabled participants to express their point of view and reflect a real world situation. Telephone interviews were used in preference to face-to-face interviews because:

- the nature of the research topic meant participants may not turn up for an interview;
- drug users may live in parts of the city which due to a high rate of crime might be considered unsafe to visit (Marcus and Crane 1986);

- the cost of undertaking telephone interviews, in terms of time, effort and money is lower (Denscombe 2003); and
- the relative anonymity of telephone interviews, lack of face-to-face contact and the establishment of confidentiality enables people to talk honestly and openly about their experiences (Carr and Worth 2001).

At a routine drug service appointment, staff offered the clients with a history of not keeping an appointment with the outreach clinic an information leaflet giving a brief explanation of the study, and invited them to participate. Those with a written or verbal diagnosis of hepatitis C (including past or current infection) or clients seeking testing were included. Clients agreeing to be interviewed were asked to complete and sign a contact details sheet giving a preferred telephone number to the researcher.

Research findings

Twenty-eight interviews were completed. For the purposes of this chapter, the findings from these interviews will focus on three areas:

(i) Beliefs and expectations about hepatitis C,
(ii) 'Bad' veins,
(iii) Poverty.

(i) Beliefs and expectations about hepatitis C

One theme emerging as important to missed appointments related to beliefs and expectations about hepatitis C (derived from different sources including other infected people). These varied and sometimes conflicted within and between participants. For example, some people felt the infection trivial and others believed there to be no effective treatment, so there was no point in turning up. Some illustrations are given here.

Asymptomatic nature of infection

There was a perception that not experiencing any symptoms of infection or that the infection is not severe and at a 'low level' meant it was reasonable not to take further action.

> . . . there is a bit of a myth what I have heard from some people that hepatitis it doesn't really matter if you have got it because it won't affect you for such a long time anyway or maybe it won't affect you at all . . .
>
> *(Male, aged <30 years old)*

Treatment: effectiveness and side-effects

For some people there was no point in attending because they mistakenly believed treatment may not cure the infection and it just makes you less infectious to other people.

Others were scared of the side-effects of treatment because they heard that people's hair falls out and so likened it to 'chemotherapy'. Some were worried about the impact of potential side-effects on their health and daily activities.

> Another thing that put me off . . . a bit as well is like treatment you know people saying to me it makes you really ill and things like that.
>
> *(Male, aged <30 years old)*

(ii) 'Bad' veins

A further explanation for missed appointments related to drug use and addiction. Sub-themes identified within this category include the physical consequences of drug use and people having 'bad' veins. People were put off keeping appointments because they anticipated staff would not get a blood sample, which also resulted in not having a clear diagnosis.

Poor experience of blood tests

People reported health professionals dismissing patients' advice of where to locate a vein, using needles that were too big and attempting several times without success.

> . . . we hate it, absolutely hate it . . . It takes ages to get any kind of blood out even a dribble and when you tell somebody where to go they'll be going . . oh no, no, no like they know best but you end up coming out looking like that thing off . . . With cotton wool balls all over us where we've been speared a million times.
>
> *(Female, aged <50 years)*

Unclear about diagnosis

Due to difficulties with getting blood, some people reported not being tested at all or they were uncertain about their diagnosis because alternative methods to blood such as mouth swabs were unable to identify whether the infection had gone or if it was still present.

> . . . I had never been tested until I'd seen P . . . till he did me that swab test in my mouth and he said it's showing antibodies but that could mean that you have had it or you have got it. I would need to go for a blood test next and that puts me off . . . there is no way I can come to you and you take blood out of me . . .
>
> *(Male, aged <40 years old)*

(iii) Poverty

The last emerging theme to explain missed appointments is poverty. People claiming benefits described the high cost of travel to services, and participants experienced difficulties in getting reimbursement of their travel expenses.

High cost of travel

Participants suggested the cost of travel to services was prohibitive, which was exacerbated if they had to attend an additional appointment in the same week, or if their usual benefit had been reduced for non-qualification of entitlement, e.g. they were subsequently deemed not sick and fit to work or because they owed the council money.

> . . . It's like expensive now on buses. It's like £5 for an all day saver and some people . . . haven't got that kind of bus fare.
>
> *(Male, aged < 40 years)*

Reimbursement of travel expenses

Whilst some people received reimbursement of their travel expenses with the drug clinic, others did not, including if they attended other agencies.

> And I think what's the point of me bloody going when I am not going to get me bus fare back.
>
> *(Female, aged < 50 years)*

In summary, people's experiences of missing appointments provided some revealing explanations, including: misperceptions and differences of opinion about the consequences of infection and its treatment; the difficulties with health professionals getting blood and not having a clear diagnosis; and being on benefits with the high cost of travel and not getting fares reimbursed.

Application to practice

From what the research participants said about missed appointments with the hepatitis C outreach clinic, it would appear that the new NICE guidance (2012b) has largely addressed the difficulties with testing they described. The guidance recognises that people at risk of infection may have poor venous access and drugs services staff need to be trained and competent to perform DBS tests as an alternative to taking blood. The participants also said that where an alternative means of testing had been used in the past, i.e. mouth swabs, a positive result only told them that they had been exposed to the infection. Thus, because a blood test was still needed to establish if the infection was present they missed an appointment and remained unclear about their diagnosis and whether they needed treatment. The new guidance (NICE 2012b) addresses the problem of an unclear diagnosis by recommending laboratories used by drug services (and other testing centres) ensure that the additional test to confirm if the infection is still present is automatically performed following an initial positive result. This policy will enable people tested at their first visit to be clear about their diagnosis and for staff to discuss referral for treatment with those chronically infected. As described under '(a) prevention of new infections', it is important that staff address the social factors which may impair people's ability to attend for treatment (Marmot 2010).

The feedback from research participants about missed appointments also identified some issues related to treatment beliefs regarding hepatitis C, such as not knowing whether it could cure the infection, if treatment was always necessary and when it should be started, whilst others had heard negative stories about its side-effects. The new testing guidance (NICE 2012b) recommends staff should have the knowledge and skills to promote treatment. Thus, the staff should then be in a position to dispel any inaccuracies or myths that people hold and inform them of the benefits of attending for specialist care and of curative treatment, despite the absence of symptoms. This research identified some of the particular issues the participants voiced about treatment, which staff should be aware of and discuss with hepatitis C infected individuals. For Marmot (2010) an early diagnosis is a priority in helping to reduce inequalities. The treatment for hepatitis C is more likely to be successful with an early diagnosis and before the development of advanced liver disease (Foster et al. 2007). In addition, following a diagnosis, people will be usually offered advice and support to make lifestyle changes to minimise further harm to the liver, e.g. reducing their alcohol intake, and to avoid infecting others by not sharing drug injecting equipment. Again, it is important that this advice and support addresses the wider social determinants of health to help people make positive lifestyle changes (Marmot 2010).

Regarding the last theme to emerge from the research, poverty, this was both a consequence of ill-health, with people being unable to gain employment, but also a determinant of ill-health, with individuals less able to access essential services (Dahlgren and Whitehead 2007). The research participants talked about the high cost of travel, which was more keenly felt as most were on benefits. Some described this problem as being exacerbated if they had to attend additional appointments or had to make choices as to how best to spend their limited income. For these reasons, it was important to the participants that they were able to get their travel expenses reimbursed, which was a difficulty for some. The new testing guidance (NICE 2012b) for drugs services recommends the possibility of providing community treatment alongside OST, which will require regular blood tests and monitoring. This, alongside the testing recommendations (including the giving of results) will create additional appointments for clients to attend. Neither the guidance nor Marmot (2010) appears to explicitly recognise the financial problems of people on low incomes having the money to attend more appointments, particularly if they are to be offered treatment. The research participants suggested services consider allocating people a monthly bus pass to help with attendance at appointments. This has been identified elsewhere to help IDUs access and benefit from services (Neale et al. 2007). Arguably this could be money well spent, as more people could be treated and cured of their infection, potentially avoiding the high healthcare costs associated with managing advanced liver disease (outlined at the beginning of the 'theory and policy' section).

Therefore it can be concluded that, when measured against findings of qualitative research into missed appointments with hepatitis C outreach clinics, the new NICE guidance (2012b) has the potential for more people to be tested for hepatitis C, and to be informed of curative treatment for which they can be referred to a specialist service. However, the qualitative research findings also indicate the guidance fails to adequately address the issue of poverty on patients' ability to keep appointments and the subsequent impact of this on their access to treatment. Addressing this issue will entail working in partnership with benefit agencies to ensure that patients are kept updated and informed of entitlement and that access to this is not complicated. This may be difficult to achieve in the context of the current climate of significant welfare benefit reform (Department of Work and Pensions 2012). Actions taken locally have included the appointment of a specialist social worker, able to broker services on behalf of patients, considering ways to reduce the number of appointments patients are asked to attend, and providing support for patients claiming their travel expenses. Thus, whilst the NICE guidance (2012b) has been successful in addressing a number of issues, from the patients' perspective it has neglected to address some of the issues which patients consider have the greatest impact on their ability or willingness to access hepatitis C testing and treatment. Had NICE used qualitative research to complement epidemiological and other quantitative research the guidance may have more fully addressed the needs of patients and arguably further reduced health inequality in the area of hepatitis C.

References

Carr, E. and Worth, A. (2001) The use of the telephone interview for research. *Nursing Times Research* 6, 1: 511–524.

Dahlgren, G. and Whitehead, M. (2007) European Strategies for Tackling Social Inequities in Health: Levelling Up Part 2. Copenhagen: World Health Organization Regional Office for Europe. Online at: http://www.euro.who.int/__data/assets/pdf_file/0018/103824/E89384.pdf Accessed September 2013.

Denscombe, M. (2003) *The Good Research Guide: For Small-Scale Social Research Projects* (2nd ed.) England: Open University Press.

Department of Health (2002) *Hepatitis C Strategy for England*. London: Department of Health.

Department of Health (2004) *Hepatitis C Action Plan for England*. London: Department of Health.

Department of Work and Pensions (2012) Welfare Reform Act 2012. Online at: https://www.gov.uk/government/organisations/department-for-work-pensions/series/welfare-reform-act-2012-impact-assessments Accessed September 2013.

Foster, G. R., Fried, M. W., Hadziyannis, S. J., et al. (2007) Prediction of sustained virological response in chronic hepatitis C patients treated with peginterferon alfa-2a (40KD) and ribavirin. *Scandinavian Journal of Gastroenterology* 42, 2: 247–255.

Health Protection Agency (2011) *Hepatitis C in the UK: 2011 Report*. London: Health Protection Agency.

Health Protection Agency (2012a) *Shooting Up: Infections among Injecting Drug Users in the UK 2011: An Update: November 2012*. London: Health Protection Agency.

Health Protection Agency (2012b) *Hepatitis C in the UK: 2012 Report*. London: Health Protection Agency.

Lewis, H., Igbe, R., Wilkinson, M., et al. (2012) Active injection drug users can be successfully treated for HCV and significantly reduce illicit drug use post treatment: Real life cohort of 152 patients. *Journal of Hepatology* 56: S446.

Long, A. (1994) Directions for Health: The Leeds Declaration. *Radical Statistics* 57: 39–42. Online at: http://www.radstats.org.uk/no057/index.htm Accessed September 2013.

Maghlaoui, A. (2012) Challenges and issues in managing hepatitis C. *Nursing Times* 108, 32/33: 18–20.

Marcus, A. and Crane, L. (1986) *Telephone Surveys in Public Health Research. Medical Care* 24, 2 (Feb): 97–112.

Marmot, M. (2010) *Fair Society, Healthy Lives: The Marmot Review.* London: The Marmot Review.

Martin, N., Vickerman, P., Foster, G., et al. (2011) Can antiviral therapy for hepatitis C reduce the prevalence of HCV among injecting drug user populations? A modelling analysis of its prevention utility. *Journal of Hepatology* 54, 1137–1144.

National Treatment Agency for Substance Misuse (2012) *Drug Treatment 2012: Progress Made, Challenges Ahead.* London: NTA.

Neale, J., Sheard, L. and Tompkins, C. (2007) Factors that help injecting drug users to access and benefit from services: A qualitative study. *Substance Abuse Treatment, Prevention and Policy* 2: 31.

NHS Choices (2012) *Hepatitis C: Get Tested. Get Treated.* Online at: http://www.nhs.uk/hepatitisc/Pages/default.aspx Accessed September 2013.

NICE (2006) *Peginterferon Alfa and Ribavirin for the Treatment of Mild Chronic Hepatitis C. NICE Technology Appraisal Guidance 106.* London: NICE.

NICE (2007) *Methadone and Buprenorphine for the Management of Opioid Dependence. NICE Technology Appraisal 114.* London: NICE.

NICE (2009) *Needle and Syringe Programmes. NICE Public Health Guidance 18.* London: NICE.

NICE (2012a) *About NICE: Who Are We.* London: NICE. Online at: http://www.nice.org.uk/aboutnice/whoweare/who_we_are.jsp Accessed September 2013.

NICE (2012b) *Hepatitis B and C: Ways to Promote and Offer Testing to People at Increased Risk of Infection. NICE Public Health Guidance 43.* London: NICE.

Shepard, C., Fineli, L. and Alter, M. (2005) Global epidemiology of hepatitis C virus infection. *Lancet Infectious Diseases* 5: 558–567.

Stephens, P. (2012) *Bridging the Gap: Why Some People Are Not Offered the Medicines That NICE Recommends.* London: IMS Health.

12

ADULTS OF WORKING AGE (AGES 25–64)

Chris Bentley

Introduction

For adults of working age, the issue of work itself, and worklessness and its consequences for standard of living, are dominant. Together with the related issues of skills development and lifelong learning, these constitute half of the priority objectives of the Marmot Review. This section of the book, and of the Life Course approach, therefore, focuses on two important components of these critical social determinants of health.

Ensure healthy standard of living for all

Policy Objective D from the Marmot Review, ostensibly about standard of living, focuses its recommendations on personal finance (The Marmot Review 2010: 187) and recommends the following:

- Develop and implement standards for a minimum income for healthy living
- Review and implement systems of taxation, benefits, pensions and tax credits to provide a minimum income for healthy living standards and facilitate upwards pathways
- Remove 'cliff-edges' for those moving in and out of work and improve flexibility of employment

The basis of the core recommendation is that if we are to achieve a healthy standard of living for all, this will require a minimum income standard that includes health needs, as well as reprioritising the tax and benefits system. Discussion moves on to the calculation of a minimum income for healthy living (MIHL). The principle takes into account the issue that, as society becomes richer, the levels of resources that are considered to be adequate also rise, otherwise the poor do not keep up with the rest of society. It is proposed that MIHL should include needs relating to nutrition, physical activity, housing, psychosocial interactions, transport, medical care and hygiene (The Marmot Review 2010: 120–121).

However, there is some inconsistency here. Much is made in the Review of the social gradient, and 'proportionate universalism'. It is not clear how this fits with the MIHL. If the gradient of life expectancy with income is fundamental, then there should be no threshold point to reach before one might expect changes. Every small increment should enable improvement, rather than there being a stepwise difference above and below the MIHL.

The reality, of course, is that, as discussed in Chapters 1 and 2 of this book, at the most deprived end of the gradient, the healthy life expectancy does fall away steeply, and becomes *disproportionate* (see Figure 2.2). Here shortfalls and disadvantages cluster, and compound each other. There may be a minimum income to help overcome these disadvantages, but it is likely that the basis of the inequalities is about more than income.

In Chapter 13, Peter Allmark explores this issue, introducing the literary debate about 'capabilities' working alongside income as determinants of a social gradient in inequality.

The chapter goes on to explore how welfare benefits and payments could actually result in health benefits. Should small increments in income resulting from welfare produce a 'proportionate' improvement in health? This does not seem to be the clear outcome. Instead there may well be variable health benefits, dependent on a range of contextual variables. His reasoned argument ranges around the use of a research tool, the logic model, which can handle diversity of positive and negative influences, in a system very different to the necessarily controlled variables of randomised controlled trials.

Create fair employment and good work for all

This Marmot Review Policy Objective (C) links closely with the objective of ensuring a healthy standard of living for all, and particularly the priority to 'remove "cliff-edges" for those moving in and out of work and improve flexibility of employment'. However, the emphasis is not just on employment at any price, but also to 'improve the quality of jobs across the social gradient' (The Marmot Review 2010: 110). This strongly echoes the core recommendation of the WHO Commission before it on Fair Employment and Decent Work (Commission on Social Determinants of Health 2008). Both refute the case that 'any job is better than no job'.

In Chapter 14 of this book, Linda Grant makes a strong case for job quality being an important public health issue. Building from the premise that there is 'robust epidemiological evidence that quality of employment has an impact on health, life expectancy and opportunity' (Coats and Lekhi 2008), she uses good qualitative research to flesh-out the meaning of the epidemiology. In particular, she draws on a large composite study, Gender and Employment in Local Labour Markets (GELLM), to explore the issues around women in part-time employment. This must be important in terms of scale alone, as millions of working age women spend much of their 30s, 40s and 50s in part-time work. If this work is poor quality, it can have a major impact on their mental, physical and spiritual health in the short and longer terms.

The Marmot working group identified ten core components of work that protect good health and promotes health (The Marmot Review 2010: 112). The challenge in relation to the public's health is whether these evidence-based practices can be systematically applied on an industrial scale, so as to make a percentage change in the population's health. Although Grant draws on international comparisons, suggesting that the UK may compare unfavourably overall in relation to job quality, GELLM findings suggest that this need not be the case. It demonstrates a variation in the availability of good part-time jobs irrespective of the industrial structure of economies. This means that individual organisations have the power to create decent jobs, independently of the context. The question for public health is how to widely replicate this good practice.

For 'sea-changes' to occur, multi-faceted approaches drawn from the Population Intervention Triangle (Chapter 2) are probably necessary. Grant and Marmot (The Marmot Review 2010: 110–115) point to possible changes in legislation, regulation and national policy as population level intervention. At service level, there are formal processes that can be improved, for example in relation to job design. At the level of the community of the workplace, much can be done in relation to informal decision making, and representation and involvement of workers in these processes. A good case can be made for the prioritisation of this issue and the application of public health knowledge, skills and techniques in an holistic approach.

References

Coats, D. and Lekhi, R. (2008) *Good Work: Job Quality in a Changing Economy*. London: The Work Foundation.

Commission on the Social Determinants of Health (2008) *Closing the Gap in a Generation*. Geneva: WHO, World Health Organisation.

Marmot Review (2010) *Fair Society, Healthy Lives*. London: The Marmot Review.

13

WELFARE RIGHTS AND THE HEALTH BENEFITS OF BENEFITS

Peter Allmark

Introduction

In many societies the wealthier are also healthier. In response, the Marmot Review recommends the establishment in the UK of a Minimum Income for Healthy Living (MIHL) in order to secure its fourth policy objective, to 'ensure a healthy standard of living for all' (Marmot 2010: 9). The report goes on to recommend establishing a minimum income for healthy living (MIHL) and an overhaul of the welfare system to make it more progressive. One implication of Marmot's recommendation is that the MIHL is not currently enjoyed by the poor in the UK. This is disputed:

> Absolute poverty in the form of an inadequate diet, overcrowding, poor hygiene and lack of protection from the elements can harm the human organism and cause disease. Relative poverty cannot.
>
> *(Le Fanu 2011: 371)*

Yet on a UK and international scale the correlation between income and health is strong and holds across the spectrum of incomes such that those on average levels of pay are less healthy than those on higher levels, and so on (Marmot 2010; Wilkinson and Pickett 2008;): this is termed a 'social gradient of health'. However, there are three puzzles here:

1. Measures that improve the financial position of the poor, such as welfare rights advice, have so far failed to show any major health effect;
2. There is a social gradient of health: health and wealth positively correlate from the poorest to the richest. This is odd: whilst we might expect those below the MIHL to have poorer health, why should this pattern persist above it?
3. The poor in relatively affluent countries are relatively poor. It is not clear why this group, who arguably have sufficient resources for a healthy life, should suffer worse

health. This puzzle deepens as some of the apparent causes of this worse health, such as higher levels of smoking or obesity, have no clear direct links to (relative) poverty. Why, for example, would the relatively poor indulge more than others in expensive and unhealthy tobacco consumption?

This chapter reports a project focused directly on the first puzzle but which has implications for the other two. The project begins with a systematic review of evidence for health effects from interventions that offer people help and advice in obtaining welfare rights and benefit payments. From this evidence, a model is constructed showing a causal chain linking the interventions to health improvements and indicating the evidential weight for each proposed link. These links suggest that the interventions have pro-health effects, that is, they tend towards improving health in the long run. They should, therefore, be viewed as health as well as social or charitable, interventions.

Theory and policy

Welfare advice and health

Some UK commissioners of local health services have pioneered the provision of advice services as part of community care. The services are sometimes provided by local government bodies but more often by charitable organisations. These advice initiatives have been funded within National Health Service provision in the expectation that such social interventions might be expected to improve recipients' health. However, an evidence review performed in 2002 and a systematic review in 2006 found little or no evidence of health benefit (Adams et al. 2006; Greasley and Small 2002). A third review in 2006 found evidence of mental health but not physical health benefit (Abbott et al. 2006). It might be argued that the improvement in finance was too small to improve health (Lundberg 2008). However, given the social gradient we would expect changes in wealth to cause changes in health; even small amounts gained through welfare benefits should make a difference.

At the end of 2010 a team including the present author undertook a different style of evidence review using an approach based methodologically in realism and involving the construction of a logic model.

Logic models versus 'black boxes'

In hierarchies of evidence for health-care interventions, randomised controlled trials are often taken to be gold-standard (Goldenberg 2006). In these, an input is tested against predicted outputs. What matters in research terms is whether the input affects outputs; what goes on in between is of less concern. This attitude is sometimes described as a 'black-box' account of theory; what goes on between input and output remains unexplored in a metaphorical black box.

The black-box approach works well where dealing with closed systems. A closed system is one in which all relevant causative elements are contained within it. In practice, no natural system is completely closed. If it were, one case would be enough to establish whether something works or not. For example, if human beings were perfectly closed systems then we would only need to see a treatment work once for us to know that it works for all. Because this is not the case, we need to look at several cases, in a trial. But by controlling the number of external (confounding) factors we can establish fairly closed, controlled, environments and establish that a treatment works to a degree of statistical confidence.

However, some environments cannot be controlled to any great extent. If we try to establish whether, for example, an information campaign reduces smoking in the UK we cannot do this in a highly controlled environment (say, a monastery of 30-year-old white Englishmen) without the results being inapplicable more widely. Social scientists need to be careful to use RCTs only where control does not render the results meaningless; it cannot be the gold standard for all studies.

The evidence reviews of welfare benefits described above took the usual route of prioritising RCT evidence. Thus they took welfare benefit advice and welfare payments to be the inputs, health improvement, the output, and the hypothesis to be tested whether the input led to the output. Their conclusion was that the hypothesis was neither confirmed nor disproved.

We took a different approach based in the realism of, for example, Pawson and Tilley (1997). Using a wide range of research data, not prioritising RCTs, we modelled what is happening inside the black box, that is, what happens between the welfare intervention and (intended) health effects. Evidence in social science is rarely unequivocal; most inputs work for some people and not for others. We might ask, for example, what works, for whom, in what circumstances. The logic model, as discussed below, can be thought of as a diagram of the black box, of what is set in motion by welfare advice and payments that can have positive health effects for some people.

The research and findings

The logic model

The research is reported elsewhere (Allmark et al. 2013) but for our purposes here the key element is the logic model, which was constructed using data derived from a review of the literature (Figure 13.1).

The model is divided into four columns. The first shows the elements of the intervention; note how wide ranging they are, something that presents a problem for RCT designs, which require the intervention to be tightly controlled and, in doing so, end up measuring an input that is unlike that ever delivered in practice. The primary outcomes, in the second column, are those that follow directly from the intervention and which are, in the main, its explicit purpose (e.g. to help with debt). The secondary outcomes, in the next column, are caused by the primary outcomes; and the tertiary outcomes, health and wellbeing, by the secondary outcomes.

The links between the columns are hypotheses or theories of causation based in the data. The strength of evidence for these links is indicated by the boldness of the line.

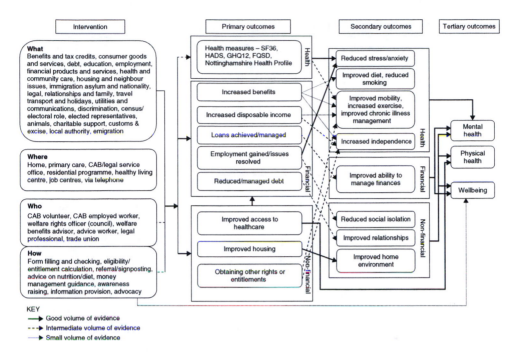

FIGURE 13.1 Logic model of potential links between advice interventions and health outcomes (Allmark et al. 2013. Reproduced with permission).

For example, the causal links to health from many of the secondary outcomes, such as reduced smoking and increased mobility, are strong. Similarly, the links between the intervention and primary outcomes such as increased disposable income are strong. Some of the links between primary and secondary outcomes are weak. For example, the link between increased benefits and reduced smoking is found only in a couple of interview studies.

If this had been a standard systematic review of evidence it would have concluded, as with previous reviews, that there was insufficient evidence to show that welfare advice either had or did not have health benefits. The logic model approach used instead was able to draw in a wider range of research, allowing links to be made with secondary and tertiary outcomes. The model shows that welfare advice sets in train pro-health mechanisms whose effects can be tracked using a range of evidence through primary, secondary and tertiary outcomes. The intervention, however, takes place in an open system such that anti-health mechanisms, such as the closure of a local employer, civil strife, welfare cuts, might negate its pro-health effects.

Mechanisms, events and experiences

The term 'pro-health' needs some explanation. Bhaskar (cited in Collier 1994) talks of three strata of reality: mechanisms, events and experiences.

TABLE 13.1 The three strata of reality: mechanisms, events and experiences

	Domain of real	Domain of actual	Domain of empirical
Mechanisms	✓		
Events	✓	✓	
Experiences	✓	✓	✓

Experiences are the phenomena, what we experience. But experience is not the whole of reality. Mechanisms operate and events occur without manifesting in empirical experiences. For example, the mechanism of gravity tends towards pushing objects downward on the Earth; and this pressure results in events in which objects are thus pushed; but numerous counter-forces might exist that prevent an empirical experience of the object falling (as when it is held up by a table, or a magnet). Gravity might be termed a pro-falling mechanism linked to events in which objects are pressured to fall and where they do fall unless another mechanism impedes that.

The same can be said of the social realm. In the logic model, health inequality and measures to reduce it (such as welfare advice) are the phenomena. The model illustrates some of the mechanisms and events triggered by the welfare advice which tend towards improving health in a way analogous to gravity tending to move objects towards earth. Whether or not objects move towards earth will depend on other factors, such as things in the way – similarly the pro-health effects of welfare advice might be countered by anti-health forces.

The pro-health effects of welfare advice

The puzzle with which the chapter began is that previous evidence reviews of research into the health effects of welfare rights advice and welfare payments have drawn a blank. By contrast, the logic model shows evidence of pro-health effects. There is strong evidence that the advice has numerous effects, such as increasing disposable income, managing debt and help with housing and with employment. And there is strong evidence that these are linked to outcomes known to improve health, such as improved home environments and reduced stress. As such, it can be said with some certainty that measures that lead to reduced stress or improved home environments will, other things being equal, improve health. There is weaker evidence that the advice links to other pro-health effects, such as improved diet and increased mobility which are also known to improve health. Again, other things being equal, these will improve health. One problem is that other things are not equal. The pro-health effects might be offset by anti-health effects, such as working in low-paid high-stress work, or losing a job.

Relative poverty and the MIHL

Let us turn now to the question of the link between relative poverty and illness. In the first place, the assertion that the poor in affluent Western societies have sufficient economic goods for health is doubtful. For example, the UK has a high level of excess winter deaths and cold-related illness largely due to people having insufficient income adequately to warm their homes. Similarly, many live in damp, overcrowded conditions known to cause health problems. It was estimated in 2009 that 3.6 million UK adults are below the MIHL (Morris et al. 2010).

This still leaves unresolved the issue of the social gradient for health which seems to persist even for those above the MIHL. One explanation, arising from the work by Wilkinson and Pickett (2008) and cited favourably in the Marmot Review, is that inequality itself damages health, and much else beside. From huge data sets they show that income inequality is associated with illness, crime, drug use, poor education and so on.

This harm–from–inequality hypothesis can be combined with the MIHL hypothesis; if both are correct we should expect a social gradient in health based on income, but with a steepening of the slope at the poorest end where people fall below the MIHL. And this is indeed what is shown in the Marmot Review's first and most celebrated graph plotting life expectancy and disability-free-life expectancy against neighbourhood deprivation. To sum up, inequality of itself causes health problems that are compounded where income falls below MIHL.

Inequality of what? The Capabilities Approach

What, though, is the mechanism by which inequality causes a social gradient in health? How is it that those above the MIHL fare less well than those even better off? Wilkinson and Pickett suggest status anxiety – people in unequal societies are stressed and rendered ill by that inequality; they might, for example, feel the need to attain material goods that are out of their current grasp. There is some psychological research supporting this, including, for example, work showing that in situations of social evaluation people experience raised levels of cortisol, which is itself linked to heart disease. However, the evidence is not overwhelming and there is some countervailing; for example, Goldthorpe (2010) suggests that it is the perception of injustice rather than inequality that causes stress; in socially hierarchical Japan there is little evidence of status anxiety. Furthermore, a little evidence suggests that some of those at the sharp end of poverty and ill-health, ethnic minority youth, do not have problems of self-esteem or status anxiety (Verkuyten 1994).

The Marmot Review hints at an alternative mechanism in its second policy recommendation: 'to enable all . . . to maximise their capabilities and have control over their lives.' (Marmot 2010) (Executive summary p. 9) The term 'capabilities' is strongly associated with the work of Amartya Sen with whom Marmot worked at the World Health Organisation; it is from this work on capabilities that we might formulate an answer to the puzzle of the social gradient.

Sen founded an approach to the theory of justice that is termed the Capability (or Capabilities) Approach (Sen 2010). The approach developed from work in the measurement of economic and social progress. The standard approach uses gross national product (GNP): on this approach, a country is making progress if, and only if, its GNP increases. This is problematic as it takes no account of:

1. distribution – a rise in GNP is compatible with continued impoverishment of many people in society;

2. unpaid domestic and other labour – for example, a rise in GNP is compatible with a loss in parents' time with children;
3. politics – a rise in GNP is compatible with dictatorship: South Africa under apartheid was the most prosperous African country but cannot be said to have been doing well;
4. other non-economic goods – a rise in GNP is compatible with a rise in ill-health, a fall in average lifespan and reduced education.

Sen's alternative to GNP is capability; what matters in assessing an economy are people's opportunities for functionings, what they can be and do. These opportunities are an individual's capability or capabilities. The to-be functionings are states such as being well nourished or not, being in a warm house or not, and being literate or not. The to-do functionings are activities such as travelling, voting, having a family life, having a rewarding job.

Which capabilities matter to all people's wellbeing such that a shortfall in them affects health and happiness? Nussbaum (2011) suggests ten capabilities that are fundamental: these include life; bodily health; bodily integrity; play; and control over one's political and material environment (see Figure 13.2).

The capabilities are incommensurable and interconnected. They are incommensurable because you cannot make up for the lack of one with more of the other; lack of bodily integrity cannot be compensated by, say, a longer life. They are interconnected because, for example, someone lacking bodily integrity is likely to have compromised health; someone with compromised health is likely to have shortened lifespan; someone who lacks affiliation will lack opportunities for play; and so on.

Relative poverty association with shortfall of capabilities

We can now return to the question of why relative poverty is associated with lifestyle-based illness, such as those due to smoking and obesity. From the capability viewpoint it could be because relative poverty of income is a marker for absolute poverty of important capabilities. The interconnectedness of capabilities means that shortfalls in capabilities cluster at the lowest end of the social spectrum; however, they can persist throughout the social gradient. For example, civil servants lower down the pecking order have less control over their work environment and may have, say, insufficient time for play. Marmot has said, citing his well-known Whitehall study of civil servants and Sen's work, that lack of control over life might be an important risk to the health of less well-off people (Marmot 2006).

Application to practice

We have presented a logic model based on a systematic review of evidence for the health effects of welfare benefits and advice; this has been linked to a broadly realist approach and to the conceptual work of Sen in relation to capabilities. What are the implications for policy and practice?

Capability	Meaning
Life	Length of life; each person's potential will differ but the point is not to have your life reduced prematurely by, for example, accident at work, starvation and so on.
Bodily health	Again, potential will differ; it is avoidable ill health that is primarily the concern of wider society, for example, that caused by malnourishment or denial of access to potentially available health care.
Bodily integrity	This term is wide-ranging but includes: the ability to move freely without (reasonable) fear of violent assault; and choice in reproduction and sexual matters.
Senses, imagination and thought	Again, wide-ranging, this capability refers to the capacities we have as animals to use the senses and as humans to think and reason. It is impaired by illness and can be inhibited by lack of education.
Emotions	To have emotions which support a flourishing human life, such as attachment and love. This is closely linked to Aristotelian notions of the role of emotions in a good life through, for example, feeling the right level of anger or fear in a situation. It can be inhibited where it is not given room to develop in childhood.
Practical reason	This is also derived from Aristotelian theory; it is the ability to reflect critically on life and to plan it to a reasonable degree; it is inhibited in political systems that deny freedom of thought and expression.
Affiliation	Human beings are social animals and cannot thrive outside society – but they can fail to thrive in social systems that, for example, cut them off from social goods on the basis of, say, race or sexual orientation. The capability to affiliate is therefore the ability to affiliate in wider society without undue fear or discrimination.
Other species	Human beings are natural beings in a natural world; this capability is one of being able to live in a good relationship with the natural world.
Play	Aristotle and Marx (amongst many others) set store in the ability of humans to live a life greater than one devoted to mere survival. Nussbaum draws on both for this capability. In Aristotle, the leisure time needed for philosophy was created by the system of slavery; Marx's vision of all humanity freed for leisure is more attractive.
Control over your environment	'Control' in this sense is relative; no-one has complete control over their political and material environment; but people lack the capability of control when they cannot play a part in the political choices affecting them and when they cannot take a fair share of the good things produced in society.

FIGURE 13.2 Nussbaum's ten capabilities.

For policy makers and public health professionals, the logic model is a device from which they can consider the case for providing welfare rights services as part of a public health programme. The first part of that case is fairly simple: such services are known to have effects that are in turn known to have positive effects (such as improved housing or reduced stress). A second part of the case is less obvious: there is some evidence that the primary outcomes of the interventions, such as improved finances, have causal links with secondary outcomes, such as improved diet or reduced smoking. It would seem worth considering combining initiatives here: rather than aim solely at people's smoking or diet, it might improve outcomes if this were combined with help with debt, housing and benefits. More broadly, such an approach seems better suited to Marmot's aim to reduce health inequalities. As mentioned in Chapter 1, many successful initiatives in public health seem to have the unwanted effect of worsening health inequalities; the relatively well-off make better use of health advice, for example. Plausibly, initiatives that combine social, financial and health interventions would avoid this.

For researchers there is specific and general application. The specific is that the logic model can direct research by showing, for example, where links in the causal chain need examining in more detail. The model may also provide the basis to develop new initiatives; one example would be combining interventions aimed at altering behaviour, such as smoking, with interventions aimed at altering circumstances, such as debt.

The general application of the model relates to those doing public health research. An approach to evidence-based medicine that gives priority to RCTs favours treatments with short causal chains in relatively closed systems (such as drugs in human bodies). Public health interventions necessarily take place in open systems and usually have long causal chains. As such, these interventions are vulnerable to the criticism that they lack a RCT-base of evidence. Public health researchers should reject this reasoning; the logic model approach is one way of reasoning differently.

References

Abbott, S., Hobby, L. and Cotter, S. (2006) What is the impact on individual health of services in general practice settings which offer welfare benefits advice? *Health and Social Care in the Community* 14, 1: 1–8.

Adams, J., White, M., Moffatt, S., Howel, D. and Mackintosh, J. (2006) A systematic review of the health, social and financial impacts of welfare rights advice delivered in healthcare settings. *BMC Public Health* 6: 81.

Allmark, P., Baxter, S., Goyder, E., Guillame, L. and Crofton-Martin, G. (2013) Assessing the health benefits of advice services: using research evidence and logic model methods to explore complex pathways. *Health and Social Care in the Community* 21, 1: 59–68.

Collier, A. (1994) *Critical Realism: An Introduction to Roy Bhaskar's Philosophy.* London: Verso.

Goldenberg, M. J. (2006) On evidence and evidence-based medicine: lessons from the philosophy of science. *Social Science and Medicine* 62, 11: 2621–2632.

Goldthorpe, J. (2010) Analysing social inequality: a critique of two recent contributions from economics and epidemiology. *European Sociological Review* 26, 6: 731–744.

Greasley, P. and Small, N. (2002) *Welfare Advice in Primary Care.* Bradford: University of Bradford School of Health Studies.

Lundberg, O. (2008) Commentary: Politics and public health – some conceptual considerations concerning welfare state characteristics and public health outcomes. *International Journal of Epidemiology* 37, 5: 1105–1108.

Le Fanu, J. (2011) *The Rise and Fall of Modern Medicine* (2nd ed.). London: Abacus.

Marmot, M. (2006) *Health in an Unequal World: The Harveian Oration*. London: Royal College of Physicians of London.

Marmot, M. (2010) *Fair Society, Healthy Lives: Strategic Review of Health Inequalities in England post 2010*. London: Department of Health. Online at: www.marmotreview.org.

Morris, J., Deeming, C., Wilkinson, P. and Dangour, A. (2010) Action towards healthy living – for all. *International Journal of Epidemiology* 39, 1: 266–273.

Nussbaum, M. (2011) *Creating Capabilities: The Human Development Approach*, Cambridge, MA: Belknap/Harvard University Press.

Pawson, R. and Tilley, N. (1997) *Realistic Evaluation*. London: Sage.

Sen, A. (2010) *The Idea of Justice*. Harmondsworth: Penguin.

Verkuyten, M. (1994) Self-esteem among ethnic minority youth in Western countries. *Social Indicators Research* 32: 21–47.

Wilkinson, R. and Pickett, K. (2008) *The Spirit Level: Why More Equal Societies Almost Always Do Better*. Harmondsworth: Allen Lane/The Penguin Press.

14

WOMEN, EMPLOYMENT AND WELL-BEING

Linda Grant

Introduction

The potential for people's employment to affect their health and well-being is firmly established in a range of research studies. Work forms a central part of many people's lives so its significance for health status gives it an important place on the public health agenda. From the perspective of the social model of health, work and the working environment are key determinants of health, with implications for both the prevention of ill health and for premature mortality and morbidity (Dahlgren and Whitehead 2007). The quality of jobs is an important dimension, as job quality can contribute to health inequalities, while good quality jobs are linked to positive health outcomes (Marmot 2010). This chapter explores a number of themes associated with the quality of employment and considers the importance for health and well-being of creating 'good work for all' (Marmot 2010: 110).

The chapter is based on research undertaken as part of a large research programme, *Gender and Employment in Local Labour Markets (GELLM)*, which entailed six different local research studies undertaken across 12 labour markets in England, as well as detailed analysis of the 2001 census and other statistical data (Yeandle 2009).[1] The specific study focused on here examined women's part-time employment. It sought to understand why, and the extent to which, women employed in part-time jobs under-utilised their qualifications, skills and labour market experience. This was a mixed method study, involving the collection and analysis of quantitative and qualitative material.

The chapter begins with a consideration of some of the relationships between health and employment. It then explores this theme further by considering the notion of 'good jobs'. What constitutes a 'good job'? Can 'good jobs' promote health? Why are 'bad jobs' a public health issue? The discussion then considers why and how poor quality part-time jobs are created and explores the implications of poor quality part-time jobs. The conclusion emphasises the importance of placing the quality of employment at the heart of the public health agenda.

Underpinning theory and policy: employment and health

The relationships between employment and health are firmly established in many research studies (Waddell and Burton 2006). When compared with unemployment and economic inactivity, employment has a positive effect on health, partly because of the income derived from work but also because of the status and social inclusion associated with employment. Indeed, this has been an important feature of the contemporary policy discourse in the context of high levels of economic inactivity (Black 2008). At the same time, the potential for work to have a negative impact on health has been evident over a long period of time. There has been a longstanding interest in health and safety at work and with workplace diseases and accidents, which sometimes lead to death or serious injury (Siegrist et al. 2010). More commonplace aspects of employment, such as low pay, long working hours, shift working and job insecurity have also featured as public health concerns (Siegrist et al. 2010). This has led to the argument that simply having a job is not enough. The quality of employment is critically important. Employees have better health when job quality is good (Constable et al. 2009; Marmot 2010), while poor quality jobs 'are more likely to make you ill' (Bevan 2012: 9–10; Coats and Max 2005: 11).

The evidence linking good quality employment to better health has been emphasised in recent policy. The *Marmot Review* (2010) is one of a number of major policy documents to highlight the significance of good quality employment for health and well-being (Marmot 2010). The Acheson inquiry also indicated the importance of job quality for health (Department of Health (DH) 1998). Even in policy proposals whose main thrust is to tackle 'worklessness', the quality of jobs is a theme (Black 2008; DH/DWP 2005). Internationally, policy published by the World Health Organisation, the European Commission and the International Labour Organisation has also focused on the significance for health of the quality of employment (Gallie 2010; Lee and McCann 2011; WHO 2008).

'Bad jobs' and 'good jobs'

Over the last decade there has been a growing interest in the promotion of good quality employment, and a discussion of the distinction to be drawn between 'good jobs' and 'bad jobs'. There are some aspects of 'bad jobs', including very low pay, long hours of work and unsafe conditions of work which, it is widely recognised, can damage health (Health and Safety Commission 2004; Siegrist et al. 2010; TUC 2010). But other, less widely acknowledged, job characteristics can be detrimental to health. 'Bad jobs' under–utilise workers' skills and qualifications, and deny workers opportunities to exercise autonomous decision-making, a theme highlighted in the major study of Whitehall civil servants undertaken by Marmot and his colleagues (see Chapter 1). In 'bad jobs' the tasks typically deny employees any discretion or control and the work is monotonous and repetitive (Coats and Lekhi 2008). Poor quality jobs are the outcome of the approach taken to job design or can derive from the wider organisation and culture of a workplace. Workplaces where managers do not acknowledge the skills of workers, treat workers without respect, or where management exercises unfair or inconsistent treatment of workers, are associated with 'bad jobs' and, in turn, with poor health (Constable et al. 2009).

There has also been a growing discussion about what constitutes good quality employment (Green 2006). 'Decent work' is advocated by the International Labour Organisation (ILO) (Lee and McCann 2011). The ILO seeks to promote opportunities for work that deliver a fair income, security in the workplace and social protection for families globally. 'Decent work' involves ensuring prospects for personal development, and freedom for people to organise amongst themselves and to participate in the decisions made at work, along with equal treatment for women and men.

In the UK, The Work Foundation has sought to promote workplace change to introduce more 'good jobs' (Bevan 2012; Coats and Lekhi 2008; Coats and Max 2005; Constable et al. 2009; Parker and Bevan 2011). 'Good jobs' allow people to use their skills and initiative and involve a variety of tasks (Gallie 2010; Green 2006; Marmot 2010). 'Good jobs' offer employees:

- employment security
- work that is not characterised by monotony and repetition
- autonomy, control and task discretion
- a balance between the efforts workers make and the rewards they receive
- the skills required to cope with periods of intense pressure
- strong workplace relationships
- the opportunity to combine work with family responsibilities
- opportunities for learning, training and progression

Creating jobs with these characteristics is important for people's experiences at work but is also critical for their health and wellbeing. Indeed, a key factor making the quality of work an important focus for policy is 'the robust epidemiological evidence that the quality of employment has an impact on health, life expectancy and opportunity' (Coats and Lekhi 2008: 14). Employment, as the social model of health emphasises, is a public health issue.

It might be argued that there will inevitably be some poor quality jobs. However, if we compare the quality of jobs in the UK with those in other, European economies it is clear that the incidence of bad jobs can be minimised. Job quality and the quality of workplace relations tend to be better in countries that prioritise job quality as a policy issue and where this forms part of the 'national conversation' (Coats and Lekhi 2008: 25; Gallie 2010). For example, in the Scandinavian countries, where job quality occupies a prominence on the policy agenda, the quality of jobs is much better (Constable et al. 2009; Gallie 2010). The strength and involvement of trade unions is a critical factor shaping the quality of employment. In the UK trade union strength is weak, and in low pay sectors and occupations trade union density is low. More importantly, in the UK trade unions are not engaged in decision-making on employment policy. Where trade unions are involved in national level decision-making on employment, as in the Scandinavian countries, this can have an important bearing on the quality of employment (Gallie 2010). In the UK, market forces are much more significant than policy in shaping the quality and levels of employment. This might explain why, although there has been growth in 'good jobs' in the British economy, the increase in 'bad jobs' with low skill content is also marked (Coats and Lekhi 2008: 24).

An important aspect of good jobs is that they can promote health and well-being (Marmot 2004; Siegrist et al. 2010). This takes the policy agenda beyond workplace health promotion or well-being schemes and practices that support sick workers to return to work, and into a consideration of the processes and practices underpinning workplace organisation and the design of jobs themselves. The health-promoting features of good jobs have been linked to the very essence of the human experience and condition. The focus with regard to quality of work is on 'the factors that contribute to the capacity for self-realization and development of employees at work rather than on the material rewards of work' (Gallie 2010: 4). Fulfilling work, in which people exercise control and judgement over the content and pace of work, and in which they apply their skills and knowledge to fulfil tasks, engenders a sense of well-being and human worth and, in turn, promotes health.

The research and its findings

The discussion that follows is based on the research undertaken for the GELLM study on women's part-time employment (Grant et al. 2005, 2006). The study undertook a survey of part-time women workers employed in 22 private and public sector workplaces in a range of industries (health, education, social care, sports, cultural services, hotels and restaurants, retail, transport and communication, food and engineering) across six localities in England (Camden, Leicester, Thurrock, Trafford, Wakefield and West Sussex). Eighty-nine part-time women workers were interviewed face-to-face, drawn from across the workplaces and chosen because they were under-using their labour market skills or qualifications in their current job. The interviews explored the reasons why they were employed 'below their potential'. Interviews were also conducted with 22 senior managers in the workplaces surveyed, exploring how and why part-time jobs were constructed, and three focus group discussions were held with 29 trade union representatives. The discussion here draws on a thematic analysis of this material, and the wider literature, highlighting themes that consistently emerged.

Bad jobs and part-time employment: a health hazard cocktail

The GELLM study revealed a strong association between poor job quality and women's part-time employment. This is significant because part-time employment is a typical form of employment for millions of women in the prime years of their working lives.

That the majority of the part-time jobs available on the open labour market are of poor quality is firmly supported by research. There are a number of dimensions to this. First, the conditions of work tend to be poor. Hourly pay is often low, access to training that would enhance progression at work is restricted, and promotion opportunities tend to be limited (Francesconi and Gosling 2005; Grant et al. 2005, 2006; Harkness 2002; Jenkins 2004; Manning and Petrongolo 2004; O'Reilly and Fagan 1998; Women and Equality Unit 2003). Secondly, typically, job content and employee autonomy are limited. Tasks tend to be repetitive, employees lack opportunities to exercise decision-making over their jobs, and flexibility with respect to hours of work and start and finish times is restricted, undermining the capacity for women to control how they combine work with family responsibilities. Thirdly, in some workplaces, part-time workers experience the negative consequence of workplace inequality. For example, they can lack the opportunities to participate in workplace decision-making offered to full-time workers, or can be derided as working 'only for pin money' (Grant et al. 2005, 2006). Fourthly, because of the dearth of good quality part-time jobs, around 50 per cent of women working in part-time jobs are working 'below their potential'. That is to say, they are employed in jobs that fail to use their skills, experience or qualifications.

> In terms of responsibility, this job is a lot more interesting than it was when I started. But, you know, I ran a company and we had about 25 staff. If there were part-time jobs that were able to use my experience it would appeal to me, but they're basically not there. I'd like a higher level of responsibility but I know that kind of job doesn't exist.
>
> *(Part-time worker, Camden)*

This finding of the GELLM research was confirmed by a follow-up survey undertaken by the Equal Opportunities Commission, which revealed that nationally 2.8 million women workers are in this situation (Darton and Hurrell 2005). The typical job occupied by a part-time woman worker is the archetypical 'bad job', with all the implications for health and well-being outlined above.

This raises the question of why good part-time jobs are not widely available on the open labour market in the UK. There are two broad sets of factors which help to explain this: formal processes of job design and informal decision-making within workplaces.

Why so few 'good part-time jobs'?

Part of the answer to this lies in informal processes within workplaces and the decisions of managers (Grant et al. 2005, 2006). In many workplaces the balance between full-time and part-time jobs remains fairly constant year on year because managers tend to replace 'like with like', part-time with part-time and full-time with full-time. Reviews of job structures, for example, when an employee leaves, are rare:

> I think over the years we've pretty much replaced like with like and we've not really thought, 'Is this role worth splitting in two?' . . . I guess no one has ever sat back and thought, 'Is there a different way of doing this?'
>
> *(Manager, Camden)*

Secondly, there can be more conscious resistance to redesigning good quality, full-time jobs as part-time. Many managers argue that the tasks involved in more senior, jobs cannot be undertaken on a part-time basis. Employing part-time workers in these jobs, it is believed, would lead to a situation where uncompleted tasks would fall to other senior post holders to complete and essential decisions would not be taken.

> It would be very difficult to justify a part-time role, say, as a duty manager . . . Where would you get the continuity in the decisions that are made? . . . You'd have to have both people doing that job in all the meetings . . . It wouldn't, it couldn't work.
>
> *(Manager, Thurrock)*

A further factor is that the costs of employing full-time and part-time workers are broadly similar but the returns for part-time workers are lower because they work fewer hours (Manning and Petrongolo 2004: 28). Managers' prejudice is also important (Tomlinson 2006). For example, there are concerns that if good quality jobs are advertised as part-time on the open labour market the calibre of candidates would be inferior.

> We are not going to get such a good field if we advertise for someone four days a week . . . The field won't be as good as it would be for full-time.
>
> *(Manager, Camden)*

Such prejudices can inform wider workplace cultures, so that part-time working and part-time workers are regarded as second best, only suitable in particular, low level jobs. Broadly, employers are reluctant to offer part-time contracts for the types of good quality jobs that are offered to full-time workers.

Why so many 'bad part-time jobs'?

A second question is why the part-time jobs typically available on the open labour market are of such poor quality. This involves a consideration of the more formal decision-making processes employers use to construct part-time jobs. The GELLM study identified some key types of part-time jobs (Grant et al. 2005, 2006). '*Task-based part-time jobs*' are based on managers' perceptions that certain tasks can be completed in a limited number of hours, e.g. cleaning an office or hospital ward, providing care to an elderly person, or offering support services to pupils in a classroom setting. Employers evaluate the length of time required to fulfil a particular task and design jobs on this basis. The aim is to use part-time employment as a means of avoiding unnecessary wage costs.

> If you're simply supporting in the classroom, as a learning support assistant, putting it bluntly, if they are not needed they are not paid . . . Obviously teachers work much longer days than that . . . With support staff we are just paying people when they need to be here.
>
> *(Manager, Camden)*

'*Demand-based part-time jobs*', such as checkout operators in supermarkets, assembly workers in manufacturing, library assistants, security workers and bar workers are designed as part-time because, employers argue, the worker is only required during a part of the working day or working week. The jobs are part-time to boost the number of workers at particular periods of high demand, providing employers with numerical flexibility (O'Reilly and Fagan 1998). Using full-time employees would not fill these gaps cost effectively. '*Recruitment-based part-time jobs*' are created to ease recruitment to low paid jobs in tight labour markets. A combination of low unemployment in a locality and the low pay offered for a specific job creates significant recruitment problems. The jobs are designed to attract women workers looking for part-time work.[2]

Because part-time jobs are created for particular reasons, this enables employers to set them apart from other jobs in the workplace or organisation. Critically, they become a self-contained group of jobs, not integrated into wider training, progression and career opportunities, offering only a narrow range of fairly repetitive tasks, and involving a high degree of monitoring and control over the worker (Grant 2009).

Superimposed on this separateness is a set of ideas that some managers use to justify the poor quality of the jobs, often revealing gendered thinking. There is an expectation that the recruits will be women, and an assumption they will be second earners.

> A typical part-time worker is somebody who has got outside commitments . . . probably supporting the family income . . . to help support the holiday and the social side of life . . . they're coming out for a bit of pocket money.
>
> *(Manager, Thurrock)*

The tasks associated with part-time jobs are regarded as quickly learned and thus the workers occupying the jobs are seen as easily replaced, 'because you are just looking for a bum on a seat' (Manager, Thurrock). The widely held but false assumption is that part-time workers are incapable of working at a higher level, unambitious and content with a low status position.

> The managers . . . have no idea of our past and they don't talk to you to find out . . . They don't tap into anything you've ever done, which is sad. It's a totally wasted resource.
>
> *(Part-time worker, West Sussex)*

Application to policy and practice

The relationship between health and employment has been high on the policy agenda in the recent period. But recent UK governments have focused on the negative effects on health of unemployment and economic inactivity, suggesting that any job is better than no job. Yet having a job is not enough to support and promote health; the quality of jobs is also critical. Simultaneously, the contemporary public health agenda has focused on individual life style choices. People have been urged to adopt healthier lifestyles: to eat well, to exercise regularly, and to refrain from smoking and drinking alcohol. While the significance of the social determinants of health is reflected in some of the major recent enquiries into health inequalities, such as *The Marmot Review*, this has not led to a practical, public health policy focus on key structures such as employment.

Consideration of the formal and informal decisions that limit the availability of good part-time jobs and create bad part-time jobs suggests genuine opportunities for public health interventions to promote 'good jobs for all'. A starting point is the development of new government policy focused on the quality of jobs, designed in collaboration with employers, workplace managers, employees and trade unions. As examples in other parts of Europe demonstrate, the 'good jobs' agenda must engage a range of key actors. Secondly, as the GELLM research showed, the creation of poor quality jobs is not inevitable; it rests on the decisions and practices of employers and managers. Employers committed to the 'good jobs' agenda, trade unions and local authorities may all have a role to play in popularising and promoting good practice in job design. Local authorities invariably have close connections with local employers; the 'good jobs' agenda could be a component of this dialogue. The basis for such developments is a much wider acknowledgement of the essential features and benefits of good jobs and the acceptance that the quality of jobs is significant for public health.

Notes

1   The programme was funded by a European Social Fund award to Professor Sue Yeandle, with match funding from 12 English local authorities, the Equal Opportunities Commission and the TUC. The GELLM research reports are available at: http://circle.leeds.ac.uk/projects/completed/labour-equalities/gellm/
2   There is another category of part-time jobs referred to as 'retention part-time jobs' by Tilly (1996). These are skilled, part-time jobs created to retain valued employees occupying senior positions and thus they are not advertised on the open labour market.

References

Bevan, S. (2012) *Good Work, High Performance and Productivity*. London: The Work Foundation.
Black, C. (2008) *Working for a Healthier Tomorrow*. London: The Stationery Office.
Coats, D. and Lekhi, R. (2008) *'Good Work': Job Quality in a Changing Economy*. London: The Work Foundation.
Coats, D. and Max, C. (2005) *Healthy Work: Productive Workplaces: Why the UK Needs More 'Good Jobs'*. London: The Work Foundation.
Constable, S., Coats, D., Bevan, S. and Mahdon, M. (2009) *Good Jobs*. London: The Work Foundation.
Dahlgren, G. and Whitehead, M. (2007) *European Strategies for Tackling Social Inequities in Health: Levelling up Part 2*. Copenhagen: WHO Regional Office for Europe.
Darton, D. and Hurrell, K. (2005) *People Working Part-Time below Their Potential*. Manchester: Equal Opportunities Commission.
DH (1998) *Independent Inquiry into Inequalities in Health Report*. The Acheson Report. London: The Stationery Office.
DH/DWP (2005) *Health, Work and Well-Being: Caring for Our Future*. London: The Stationery Office.
Francesconi, M. and Gosling, A. (2005) Career paths of part-time workers. EOC Working Paper Series no. 19, *Working below Potential: Women and Part-Time Work*. Manchester: Equal Opportunities Commission.
Gallie, D. (2010) *Employment Regimes and the Quality of Work*. Oxford: Oxford University Press.

Grant, L. (2009) Job design and working hours: key sources of gender inequality. In S. Yeandle (ed.) *Policy for a Change: Local Labour Market Analysis and Gender Equality*. Bristol: The Policy Press.

Grant, L., Yeandle, S. and Buckner, L. (2005) *Working below Potential: Women and Part-Time Work*. Working Paper Series no. 40. Manchester: Equal Opportunities Commission.

Grant, L., Yeandle, S. and Buckner, L. (2006) *Working below Potential: Women and Part-Time Work: Synthesis Report*. GELLM Series 2 Part 2. Sheffield: Centre for Social Inclusion, Sheffield Hallam University.

Green, F. (2006) *Demanding Work: The Paradox of Job Quality in the Affluent Economy*. Princeton and Oxford: Princeton University Press.

Harkness, S. (2002) *Low Pay, Times of Work and Gender*. EOC Research Discussion and Working Paper Series, Manchester: Equal Opportunities Commission.

Health and Safety Commission (2005) Health and Safety Commission Annual Report and the Health and Safety Commission/Executive Accounts 2004/05. London: The Stationery Office.

Jenkins, S. (2004) Restructuring flexibility: case studies of part-time female workers in six workplaces. *Gender, Work and Organization* 11, 3: 306–333.

Lee, S. and McCann, D. (eds) (2011) *Regulating for Decent Work: New Directions in Labour Market Regulation*. Geneva: International Labour Organisation.

Manning, A. and Petrongolo, B. (2004) *The Part-Time Pay Penalty*. Report for the Women and Equality Unit. London: Department of Trade and Industry.

Marmot, M. (2004) *Status Syndrome: How Your Social Standing Directly Affects Your Health and Life Expectancy*. London: Bloomsbury.

Marmot, M. (2010) *Fair Society, Healthy Lives. The Marmot Review: Strategic Review of Health Inequalities in England post-2010*. Online at: www.ucl.ac.uk/marmotreview Accessed September 2013.

O'Reilly, J. and Fagan, C. (1998) *Part-Time Prospects: An International Comparison of Part-Time Work in Europe, North America and the Pacific Rim*. London: Routledge.

Parker, L. and Bevan, S. (2011) *Good Work and Our Times: Report of the Good Work Commission*. London: The Work Foundation.

Siegrist, J., Benach, J., McKnight, A., Goldblatt, P. and Muntaner, C. (2010) *Employment Arrangements, Work Conditions and Health Inequalities*. Report on new evidence on health inequality reduction, produced by Task Group 2 for the Strategic Review of Health Inequalities post 2010.

Tilly, C. (1996) *Half a Job: Bad and Good Part-Time Jobs in a Changing Labour Market*. Philadelphia, PA: Temple University Press.

Tomlinson, J. (2006) Women's work–life balance trajectories in the UK: reformulating choice and constraint in transitions through part-time work across the life-course. *British Journal of Guidance and Counselling* 34, 3: 365–382, doi: 10.1080/03069880600769555.

TUC (2010) *In Sickness and in Health? Good Work and How to Achieve It*. London: TUC.

Waddell, G. and Burton, K. (2006) *Is Work Good for Your Health and Well-Being?* London: The Stationery Office.

WHO (2008) *Closing the Gap in a Generation: Health Equity through Action on the Social Determinants of Health*. Geneva: World Health Organisation.

Women and Equality Unit (2003) *Individual Incomes of Men and Women 1996/7 to 2001/2*. London: DTI.

Yeandle, S. (ed.) (2009) *Policy for a Change: Local Labour Market Analysis and Gender Equality*. Bristol: The Policy Press.

15

ADULTS OF RETIREMENT AGE (65+)

Chris Bentley

Introduction

At this end of the 'Life Course', the Marmot Review registers the impact of an accumulation of positive and negative impacts of the social determinants affecting the state of health and wellbeing. However, there is still plenty that can be done to address inequality and support Healthy Lives in the post-retirement period (The Marmot Review 2010:176). The following two projects provide illustrative examples of this.

The little society: collaborative working with the voluntary sector and the NHS

Right across the social gradient, older age can trigger health and social inequalities. As partners and friends pass away, loneliness and isolation can become huge issues for wellbeing. These can be compounded by physical illness and disability, and particularly by mental illness. Depression, affecting up to 16 per cent of the over 65s, and dementia, affecting around a third of people by the age of 90, are common, and on the increase. In addition, there are many people with long-standing psychotic illness, such as schizophrenia and others with late-onset mental health problems such as delirium (Mental Health Foundation 2013).

The Marmot Review recommends two critical types of intervention relevant to the development of healthy and sustainable places and communities to support the needs of older people:

*   Integrate local delivery systems to address social determinants of health
*   Improve community capital and reduce social isolation.

Linked programmes which address both of these issues, and more, are the basis of the evaluative research project covered by Nick Pollard in Chapter 16. The study itself is a small one that focuses on an often overlooked group, that is, those with complex and chronic mental health problems. It illustrates a number of critical issues very well, pointing the way towards the need to scale up such programmes across communities and, at best, society.

The programme described is a perfect illustration of activity at the base of the Population Intervention Triangle; 'service engagement with the community' (see Chapter 2). Here the voluntary and community sector has grown out of the community which it serves, and through two components described as 'the Project' and 'the Allotment' can offer 'life-saving' environments which are much valued by very needy, and previously desperate individuals. The links into service have been cemented by the enlightened 'Northside' General Practice, who partly commission the programme. This action was based on good needs assessment, recognising the increased numbers of people with chronic mental health needs, partly due to the proximity of the practice to a former 'asylum'. The needs identified were, in medical terms 'low-level', but in social wellbeing terms, critical. The integration of disparate services established by this connectivity, however, revolutionised the ease of access in both directions.

The programme itself has produced a 'sea-change' in the lives of the people it has engaged with. It would not, on its own, register a percentage change at population level. However, it appears to be cost effective, and sustainable. Testament to this is the interviewee who was very happy to pay a contribution himself with his personalised budget for attendance. He would not be without it, unlike the untailored, more formal social care arrangements previously offered. If 'small-is-beautiful' programmes sharing these characteristics became widespread, they could potentially, together, have positive impacts adding up to an industrial scale. Enlightened commissioning and planning of public health, such as 'Northside', could promulgate the expansion of such needs-based small-scale developments through their own commissioning plans within the local Health and Wellbeing Strategy.

Keeping warm and well in later life

As identified earlier in this book, ensuring a healthy standard of living for all requires more than a minimum income for healthy living (Chapter 13). There is also an important component of 'capabilities' which comes into play. Knowledge, skills, experiences, values, beliefs and expectations accumulated across the Life Course will all have an impact on standards of health and wellbeing achieved in older age.

This is well illustrated by Angela Tod in Chapter 17 as she addresses another specific Marmot Review issue around 'healthy and sustainable places'. The recommendation to 'reduce fuel poverty' applies across the age groupings, but is particularly relevant to older people (The Marmot Review 2010: 133–134). The KWIILT project, as described, was able to produce well validated qualitative data from older adults and a variety of service providers, and to combine this with temperature measurements within the homes. Analysis of this information produced a clustering or 'segmentation' of the older population sample into six distinct groups. To illustrate these groupings a pen-portrait was developed for each of the six 'types', enabling them to be used together as a working model to explore the possible consequences of the findings for practical action. One of a number of important findings was that not all of the households living in cold homes were 'fuel poor'. A proportion of the sample could probably afford to heat their homes, but for a range of reasons explored in the chapter, ended up not doing so.

This issue as described provides a good illustration of the 'Decay Model' outlined in Chapter 2 of this book. Interventions to address cold damp housing, as Tod describes, have the potential to reduce a proportion of seasonal excess deaths and illness in England caused finally by diseases of the chest and heart. However, only a proportion of those who might benefit do so. The KWIILT study provides valuable information to help calibrate all four components of the model, so that strategies can be developed to maximise the potential of the warm-home intervention:

A. *Knowledge and understanding*: About the risk of cold; about myths, what can be done?
B. *Presentation and case-finding*: Identifying those at risk; how and by whom? What will persuade them to come for help? Where will they be prepared to engage?
C. *Service effectiveness and quality*: What makes a user-friendly service? How effective and cost effective are the solutions perceived to be?
D. *Support for self-management*: What will it take for any offered solution to be used effectively by the householder? Involvement in the decisions? Training and support? After 'sales' service?

One of the key findings from the KWIILT research is that the answers, and certainly the combination of answers, to these questions are likely to be different for each of the six groups. This is critical, because unless the approaches are tailored appropriately to the characteristics of segmental groupings such as these, the outcomes achieved are unlikely to add up to change at population level.

References

Marmot Review (2010) *Fair Society, Healthy Lives*. London: The Marmot Review.
Mental Health Foundation (2013) *Older People*. Online at: http://www.mentalhealth.org.uk/help-information/mental-health-a-z/O/older-people/Accessed August 2013.

16

THE LITTLE SOCIETY

The personalisation agenda and sustaining older adults with enduring mental health needs in community care provision

Nick Pollard

Introduction

There is a lack of in-depth understanding of the experiences and needs of people with severe and complex mental health problems. This chapter draws on a realistic evaluation (Pawson and Tilley 2003) of two public health interventions examining the significance of voluntary groups in supporting a vulnerable group of older adults. In order to provide focused insight, and capture the reality of patients' experiences, it includes insights from subsequent interviews with two patients with self-directed service budgets.[1] Studies in the UK and other countries (Bryant et al. 2010; Connell et al. 2012) have identified that a combination of socio-economic and community factors, some within and some beyond the control of clinical staff, can affect quality of life for older adults with severe and complex mental health problems. The chapter will explore some of these social factors and discuss findings that suggest the value of sustained low key activities as a basis for community support.

The author is particularly grateful to the participants and the support of the partner organisations in facilitating meetings. To protect the anonymity of the participants pseudonyms have been used. 'Northside' is the project location, a very culturally diverse area with some of the lowest deprivation scores in England. A doctor's surgery together with its local partners were involved in delivering the interventions, referred to here as 'the Project' and 'the Allotment'. They form part of a pattern of flexible services and horticultural and creative pursuits as key community activities of people with severe or complex mental health problems.

Underpinning theory and policy

The Marmot Review (2010) indicated the relationship between social and economic factors which have a cumulative effect on health disparities. People with severe and enduring mental illnesses who are over 65 have often experienced a lifetime of low expectations of employment and low income, a greater risk of smoking and reduced opportunities for good diet or exercise, the effects of medication regimes, and the long term consequences of associated depression and anxiety that accompany psychiatric disorders. Amongst its objectives, the review recommended that people have the opportunity for greater control over their lives, with better information, monitoring and service delivery concerning health outcomes.

Previous government policy had recognised the need for fairer access to social care services (Department of Health [DH] 2003), yet at the same time for service restrictions in the face of increasing demand. The Government document *Putting People First* (HM Government 2007) set out service reforms for tighter eligibility with stronger local community support. An emphasis on preventative measures for the maintenance of health (DH 2008a, 2008b, 2009a, 2009b) was intended to increase opportunities for a widening range of providers, including social enterprise and charities, to be involved in delivering services (Marks and Hunter 2007). Subsequent government policy (enshrined in the Health and Social Care Act 2012) emphasised the delivery of mental health services by social firms, charities and other providers, contracted by clinical commissioning groups,[2] of which general practitioners were to be the core.

In the UK the majority of people with severe and complex mental health problems live in the community and are cared for by their local general practitioners, based in primary care practices. Burns and Kendrick's (1997) study found that primary care practices within three miles of a psychiatric hospital tend to have higher concentrations of patients with chronic mental illnesses than those in other areas. This suggests that people living in the community with severe and complex needs tend to cluster near psychiatric facilities.

When local asylum patients were relocated to the community in the 1980s and 1990s, the relatively affordable large Victorian houses of 'Northside' were converted into private nursing homes. By the early 1990s general practitioners and an occupational therapist working at a local surgery identified 100 patients with psychotic conditions (Cook and Howe 2003; Cook et al. 2004). According to one of the doctors, they found a group of

> . . . stable people who were not making a lot of fuss, they were not getting any input and they were just sitting there quietly mouldering, and they had all their medical problems as well, which weren't being looked at.
>
> *(Dr 4)*

Consequently, the Project was set up in partnership with the medical practice to develop community based services in 1993. By 2010, the practice had 126 patients with diagnoses of schizophrenia, bipolar disorder and other psychoses. The Allotment began in 1999 within the Project, but has since become a stand-alone charitable organisation. Both work with service users or 'members' who do not easily engage with statutory services. They include people from some of the cultural minorities living nearby, including asylum seekers. Some of the Projects' core service objectives concern meeting 'the physical, social and psychological needs of adults and older adults with mental health problems'. Its workers and volunteers promote recovery, integration and social inclusion, providing care programme co-ordination to individuals with severe and enduring mental health problems who do not engage with statutory services, supporting individuals and their families, and working with local primary care, voluntary, private and statutory services.

Continued changes in NHS services (Department of Health 2008a) have reduced access to services for marginalised communities and community members, who often experience complex and multiple health issues combined with communication problems. As the policy came into effect, both projects lost some funding and had to scale back their programmes; at the time of writing this chapter the Allotment was about to resume its former level of activity. Personalised budgets for self-directed services (DH 2009b, 2010) had enabled some members to find new ways to meet their care needs through the Allotment.

The research and its findings

Methods

The evaluation was funded on a small grant from NHS Sheffield. Building on earlier research (Cook and Howe 2003; Cook et al. 2004) this evaluation involved focus groups with members of the two projects, interviews with two general practitioners and two project workers, and questionnaires based on interview questions which were made available to everyone involved in the project (Pollard and Cook 2012). Follow-up interviews were conducted two years later with two of the older members to provide insight into individual trajectories for older participants regarding health needs and the impact of self-directed support. It was difficult to find older people with these needs who were using the service and willing to be interviewed. One agreed if supported by a project worker. The service evaluation was approved by Sheffield Hallam University. Numbered codes assigned to the quotes are used to distinguish different participants prefaced by an indication of whether they were a doctor (Dr) or member (M). The majority of quotes come from the older interviewees M1 and M2.

Impact of the projects

The projects provide structure to people who would otherwise, often by their own admission, not be enabled to take part in meaningful activities, develop social relationships or make a demand on services. They use media such as horticulture, arts and craft and other activities as vehicles for modelling social relationships which facilitate an experience of personal regard for the individual. One member reported that it was important that

> we're nurtured as people, because all of us for different reasons have had rubbish in our lives.
>
> *(M13)*

One older member explained how his problems had only been diagnosed after a lifetime of mental health problems and isolation. For most of his life he lived with a parent for whom he became a carer, and who died a few years ago. He left his last job in the 1980s following a disagreement. He described his routine:

> Much of the day I'm sat listening to the radio or the telly. I do potter about. A lot of the time I just do nothing. I do have time to tidy up and that, but it just ticks slowly. [. . .] A lot of the time I just get myself down, I'm hoping I'll get myself out of it in time.

Although he can cook, 'cleaning the kitchen – I think I'll do them later. Then I get an infection of flies' (M1).

Attending the Allotment one day a week helped to structure his time, and introduced him to new activities such as chair–aerobics and learning a musical instrument. The consequences of some of his behaviours had made him anxious about going into the town centre.

The partnership recognised that various activities which were once provided at the Asylum, including a farm and gardens as well as other low key occupations, were 'a missing piece' in the engagements offered to people with enduring mental health problems. One doctor explained that

> . . . the old fashioned things that used to happen in places like the Asylum have been a very low priority. And I think that we've been ahead of the game by putting them back in again and it's only now that perhaps the NHS/psychiatry services have realized that there's a large role for activity based work with people. So that's the 'Project', and I'd say the Allotment has been fantastic in maintaining people through having an open door process.
>
> *(Dr 3)*

Longevity and caring relationships

The general practitioners reported that the close relationship between their practice and the two organisations enabled more effective management of members' health. Problems could be quickly identified and neglect prevented. But, some of the relationship was less directly related to traditional perspectives of health, and more about wellbeing:

> We're getting people to look at things in a different way and separate practical and pragmatic service that has very little to do with me looking at people's diagnoses and prescriptions and that part of their care. That's very healthy.
>
> *(Dr 3)*

Members also suggested that long term relationships with staff and the project's continuity had contributed to increases in their confidence, or else noted that they had not needed to see their general practitioners as often. Some members had described how they felt valued through the personal contact made with them by the project workers. One member described the importance of having a place where he can address his anxieties:

> . . . to actually go to bed at night with the sort of feeling that it's desperate, you've got problems and you don't know what's going on tomorrow, [. . .] – it's an awful place to be in, but when you go to bed at night and you can think 'I'll let that go for a bit, and tomorrow I'll speak to someone about how much it's affecting me' it's really good.
>
> *(M1)*

Significantly, despite lifelong histories of mental health problems, social isolation, experiences of stigmatisation, and considerable personal difficulties, participants found the structure of the activities provided by the two organisations valuable in enabling their social engagement, developing activities and enjoying friendships. One was able to make friendships and be valued in a world of very few friends; for another, it was important to have space to talk about and work through his own issues. He remarked of his problems:

> . . . that seems to have like slowly gone, much calmer. Now all I want to do is enjoy whatever it is that's coming to me at the moment.
>
> *(M2)*

The other interviewee, trying out a wider range of activities, felt 'I've got more friends than I ever had' (M1).

The impact of personalised budgets

The above participant needed reassurance that he was competent to manage his own finances or household tasks. He received £183 a week in benefits, and decided to apply for personal budgeting monies to maintain a place at the Allotment. However, he needed support from his support worker with the 34-page form which included sections on 'managing my actions' and 'making decisions and organising my life':

> It has been hard work, it has been exhausting. Some of the questions were very difficult, just thinking what's the best answer, it was quite daunting.
>
> *(M1)*

He and his support worker agreed to disagree where the questions touched on issues about which he had to reflect, such as having someone to facilitate him in managing aspects of his behaviour that he had not understood would cause problems with others in the surrounding community.

Personal budgeting has not proved to be helpful for another member, who had experienced bipolar disorder for over 30 years. Despite some admissions to hospital, he had managed to stay in work until retirement. As his job had a good pension scheme he had a lump sum, which he simply left in the bank. Then

> about a year ago I had this form and it was from social services [. . .] eventually it came out that I'd be given a budget to work on and with what I'd got in the bank

from retirement and my house and everything else I wouldn't get a penny and everything that I was getting support from apart from the Allotment would have to be paid for. [. . .] I was going to be asked to pay for everything regardless of whether I thought it would be beneficial to me.

(M2)

Non-residential personal support was entirely self-funded if an individual had capital of over £23,250 (Sheffield City Council 2012b). He was sceptical about the value of the groups he was being offered as support, such as wellness therapy. He gave his perspective of a socialisation group which involved

an afternoon session, where we'd turn up at one o'clock on a Friday afternoon, and we'd go to the pictures, or shopping or whatever. [. . .] I was having these panic attacks [. . .], they'd rush off to the shops and that and I'd be sat in a park somewhere hoping that they'd come back and we could go back on the bus. I'd have these terrible feelings that I needed to go to the toilet and we're on the bus and it's a nightmare but there was nothing I could do about it and I'd got nothing to chat about because everybody was supposed to be focused on either going to the pictures or going shopping but don't talk about your personal problems because that's not what we're here for. [. . .] It might cost me £50 or £60 for an afternoon going out like that [. . .] It took a lot of doing but I did say that no I can't do this, it's not cutting right. I'd got to the stage where that money is mine, and I'd like to have a big say in how I deal with it.

(M2)

This member opted out of self-directed services, as clearly his needs were not being met in these situations.

I spoke to the psychiatrist about it and he could see my point what I was trying to get over. I do pay for things at the Allotment now but I think it's worth its weight in gold, [. . .] I'm getting a lot out of it.

(M2)

Application to practice

The evaluation indicates how the projects met needs that the statutory services did not provide. There was a continuous need to support vulnerable people to develop sustained community engagements at their own pace of adjustment, and this required some distinct processes involving activity and maintaining contact. Pressure to move on to other services is inappropriate to preventing the development of more chronic illness and depression. This data highlights the importance of a service which offers support, for example, where there is potential for problem behaviours to be misinterpreted and precipitate someone into a crisis if left alone and isolated. An illustrative hypothetical example might be someone with an engrossing interest in public transport vehicles who trespassed into bus garages to obtain photographs of rare buses and related vehicles like breakdown tractors. The individual may think they are doing no harm because in earlier decades, and perhaps in their own experience, these activities would have been more easily tolerated. A greater perception of risk has changed that. People taking pictures of buses have been challenged by concerned policemen and members of the public (Palmer and Whyte 2010). In these situations a vulnerable person might both react and be dealt with inappropriately.

Managing such issues requires the kind of trusting relationship which is built from workers and members over time. An important finding concerned the longevity of these services. This meant that referrers perceived them as reliable and anticipated a positive outcome from referrals. Members reported improved confidence, wellbeing and self-esteem from access to services over time.

Locality was an important element of this contact. The sustainability of the projects, their ability to link in and make use of other sources depended on the fostering of a community spirit and the maintenance of a mutual regard between all those involved. This appears to confirm some of the objectives of the Marmot Review (2010): the project itself had developed out of local knowledge of the particular community. The interviews with members described experiences of considerable anxiety or panic attacks, with social isolation and a degree of vulnerability linked to these symptoms that makes travel across the city or the use of public transport difficult. There was less incentive to engage with services located further away if the benefits they provide are not clear to the patient.

These kinds of issues are addressed in some of the statements and assessments in the personal budgeting process. They are implied by the assessment form questions about being part of the community and making decisions and organising one's life (Sheffield City Council 2012a), reflecting some of the issues raised by the Marmot Review, but the form they take is expressed in a functional way. The Marmot Review, with its evocation of Neruda's *The Captain's Verses*, implies a more passionate engagement with human values, and states clearly that social indicators of health might be more significant to communities and society than the pursuit of economic growth. People with chronic psychiatric disorders are a particular indicator of the extent of health inequalities. The economist Max-Neef (2010: 206) has set out human needs and values which are not materially quantifiable. Across the dimensions of 'needs, being (qualities), having (things), doing (actions), and interacting (settings)', these include 'satisfiers' such as the expression of being through 'respect, tolerance, sense of humour, generosity, sensuality', which can take place in settings such as 'intimate spaces for togetherness' and offer opportunities to 'co-operate', 'take care of', 'develop awareness', 'be different from'. Such human values, he suggests, predated money, and are therefore more fundamentally important. They are not, unlike financial values, seen as independent, operating on economic principles which are divorced from social effects, but are interrelated. They are the underpinning elements of the experience of a quality of life, and in the light of both the Francis Report (2013) and the issues such as belonging, identified by Connell et al. (2012), of care.

At 65 years of age, people with severe and complex mental health problems may have lost family and be isolated in the community. Services may not provide for their specific needs, and if they find that they are ineligible for financial support they may withdraw from them. The evaluation provides insight into how the Allotment and the Project have introduced and supported members to a range of experiential opportunities, to find the means to finance their attendance by enabling them to negotiate their choices, and maintained their connection to a primary health care service. This is enabled by a basis in an informal, low key range of activities, an emphasis on personal approaches to care, and realistically achievable goals for members. In effect, what is produced is a model of a little society, which operates within a wider community. Its principles allow people to feel at ease with each other and the people they work with.

Local and accessible resources and a community ethos enable the Project and the Allotment to facilitate their members in independent engagement with other community organisations. Members are, largely, positive about their lives, enjoy participating in healthy activities, social networks, and even taking up new pursuits. As the population ages and more people join this group the voluntary agencies attached to 'Northside' may find it useful to explore their cost-effectiveness and the sustainability of this bespoke approach to managing the needs of older people with long term mental health needs as a model for future developments.

Notes

1   Self-directed service budgets were phased into practice from 2007. People who are eligible for social care support can apply to be assessed for a personalised budget to meet their needs. Eligible people can apply to manage the budget themselves or have others manage it for them. The budgets are operated by local councils and their flexibility varies between different authorities.
2   Clinical commissioning groups were established in 2012. They include all the general practitioners (i.e. primary care doctors) in a local area and liaise to organise healthcare services with local authorities, hospitals and other health and social care professionals.

References

Bryant, W., Vacher, G., Beresford, P. and McKay, E. (2010) The modernisation of mental health day services: participatory action research exploring social networking. *Mental Health Review Journal* 15, 3: 11–21.

Burns, T. and Kendrick, T. (1997) Care of long-term mentally ill patients by British general practitioners. *Psychiatric Services* 48, 12: 1586–1587.

Connell, J., Brazier, J., O'Cathain, A., Lloyd-Jones, M. and Paisley, S. (2012) Quality of life of people with mental health problems: a synthesis of qualitative research. *Health and Quality of Life Outcomes* 10: 138 http://hqol.com/content/10/1/138.

Cook, S. and Howe, A. (2003) Engaging people with enduring psychotic conditions in primary mental health care and occupational therapy. *British Journal of Occupational Therapy* 66, 6: 236–246.

Cook, S., Howe, A. and Veal, J. (2004) A different ball game altogether: staff views on a primary mental healthcare service. *Primary Care Mental Health* 2: 77–89.

Department of Health (2003) *Fair Access to Care Services: Guidance on Eligibility Criteria for Adult Social Care*. London: DH.

Department of Health (2008a) *High Quality Care for All, NHS Next Stage Review*. London: Department of Health.

Department of Health (2008b) *The Operational Framework 2009/10*. London: Department of Health.

Department of Health (2009a) *The NHS Constitution, the NHS Belongs to Us All.* London: Department of Health.

Department of Health (2009b) *Transforming Community Services, Enabling Patterns of Provision.* London: Department of Health.

Department of Health (2010) *Prioritising Need in the Context of Putting People First: A Whole System Approach to Eligibility for Social Care.* London: Department of Health.

Francis, R. (2013) *Report of the Mid-Staffordshire NHS Foundation Trust Public Inquiry.* London: HM Stationery Office.

Health and Social Care Act 2012. Online at: http://www.legislation.gov.uk/ukpga/2012/7/contents/enacted Accessed September 2013.

HM Government (2007) *Putting People First: A Shared Vision and Commitment to the Transformation of Adult Social Care.* London: HMG.

Marks, L. and Hunter, D. J. (2007) *Social Enterprises and the NHS Changing Patterns of Ownership and Accountability.* London: Unison.

Marmot Review (2010) *Fair Society, Healthy Lives.* London: The Marmot Review.

Max-Neef, M. (2010) The world on a collision course and the need for a new economy. *Ambio* 39: 200–210.

Palmer, D. and Whyte, J. (2010) 'No credible photographic interest': photography restrictions and surveillance in a time of terror. *Philosophy of Photography* 1, 2: 177–195.

Pawson, R. and Tilley, N. (2003) *Realistic Evaluation.* London: Sage.

Pollard, N. and Cook, S. (2012) The power of low-key groupwork activities in mental health support work. *Groupwork* 22, 3: 7–32.

Sheffield City Council (2012a) Assessment Questionnaire for a Personal Budget. SCC Version 7.00. Online at: https://www.sheffield.gov.uk/caresupport/adult/how-get-support/assessment.htn Accessed September 2013.

Sheffield City Council (2012b) Information about Contributions for Non-residential Support. Online at: https://www.sheffield.gov.uk/caresupport/adult/how-get-support/costs-to-you/chargesnonrescare.html#supportnotpay Accessed September 2013.

17

KEEPING WARM AND WELL IN LATER LIFE

Angela M. Tod

Introduction

Being cold at home places people at considerable risk of physical and mental ill health and has a negative impact on wellbeing (Marmot Review Team 2011). For some, risk is heightened, for example, for the old, very young, those with pre-existing ill health and those in financial hardship. Living in a cold home could be both a cause or effect of factors identified in all of the key objective areas outlined in *Fair Society, Healthy Lives* (Marmot Review 2010; and see Table 1.1 of this volume). In terms of policy recommendations, Marmot focuses on reducing fuel poverty in each of the five life course stages Marmot Review (2010). However, whether someone is able to keep warm will depend on many and complex inter-relating factors of which fuel poverty is only one factor. This chapter reflects on selected findings from research that focuses on older people's experiences and struggles to keep warm at home, the Keeping Warm in Later Life projecT or KWILLT.[1]

The evidence of traditional epidemiological data has told us how many people are in fuel poverty or succumb to excess winter deaths. A proportion of these events will be related to older people being cold at home (Department of Health 2012a, 2012b). However, this type of epidemiological data is limited in helping us to understand *why* older people are unable to keep warm at home, and how extrinsic, contextual issues like income, housing and health, interrelate with more subtle intrinsic, social and cultural influences. In order to understand this complex picture qualitative methods are required. KWILLT aimed to use qualitative approaches to generate the insight necessary to understand older people's heating behaviour and decisions and so better understand how to overcome associated barriers.

Underpinning theory and policy

Older people and cold homes: a public health hazard

Every year there are an average of 25,100 excess winter deaths (EWDs) in England and Wales (Department of Health 2012b). EWDs are derived from deaths in the winter period (December to March) compared to the number of deaths that occurred in the preceding and following months. EWDs occur predominantly in those over 75 (Office of National Statistics 2012), due to increased rates of chronic ill health and co-morbidities (such as cardiovascular and respiratory conditions), restrictions on mobility, and less body fat to retain heat (Department of Health 2011). These factors also put older people at risk of cold-related illness, as well as death.

Other issues that put some older people at risk of the negative health impacts of being cold at home include living alone in a home that was once lived in by a family. In their solitude some older people struggle to afford heating or maintain the energy efficiency of a home. Also, around half the households in fuel poverty are lived in by people over 60 (Department of Health 2011). The current UK definition of fuel poverty is if a household needs more than 10 per cent of the total income to afford to heat the home to World Health Organisation safe temperatures (18° in the bedroom and 21° in the living room). Three factors are used to explain fuel poverty: the energy efficiency of the property, cost of fuel and income of the house. Being in fuel poverty means older people are more likely to experience exacerbations of existing illness or new health problems due to being cold (Marmot Review Team 2011).

The policy agenda

Older people may be vulnerable to the negative health impact of cold because of mental or physical illness, social isolation, having limited mobility, fuel poverty and struggling on a pension or 'flat' income. The public health importance of these issues is highlighted in the UK in the Public Health Outcomes Framework (PHOF) (Department of Health 2013) and the Cold Weather Plan (CWP) for England (Department of Health 2011, 2012a). Fuel poverty was included in the PHOF as an outcome necessary in addressing wider determinants of health, whilst EWDs was selected as a focus for healthcare provision to avoid premature mortality. The Cold Weather Plan (Department of Health 2012a,b) sets down a series of steps, actions and responsibilities for the NHS, local authority, other public sector and voluntary organisations, frontline staff and communities in preventing harm and addressing health risk from cold weather.

In understanding why some older people are cold at home, the broader policy agenda is important to consider. As well as health, other policy initiatives such as energy, housing and welfare are all undergoing fundamental reform as this chapter is being written. Alongside policy changes to affordable warmth support, additional policy innovations include changes to housing benefit, welfare reform and higher energy and fuel taxation. It is unclear how the individual and combined impact of these policies will play out in terms of fuel poverty, cold-related harm and vulnerable groups being able to keep warm.

Keeping Warm In Later Life projecT (KWILLT)

The project that is the focus of this chapter, KWILLT, aimed to provide some insight into the extrinsic factors (such as fuel cost, income and housing) and intrinsic factors (such as beliefs, attitudes and values) influencing and constraining vulnerable older people in keeping warm in their home. Also explored were the barriers and obstacles in keeping warm.

KWILLT used the theory of lay epidemiology and use of lay knowledge in decision making related to health behaviours as a framework for the study (Davison et al. 1991, 1992; Frankel et al. 1991). "Lay epidemiology" is a term used to describe the processes through which health risks are understood and interpreted by lay people, and then how these influence behaviour. According to lay epidemiology empirical beliefs about the nature of illness are recognised as important but so also are the values people have about health and risks to health in a good life. Lay epidemiology seeks to understand why people behave as they do, even if this contradicts public health messages based on traditional epidemiological data, thus embracing the principles of the Leeds Declaration (see Chapter 1). This is important in public health as both elements have to be dealt with if schemes or programmes are to be successful in promoting and supporting healthy behaviour, in this case keeping warm at home (Allmark and Tod 2006).

The chapter now focuses on lack of information and knowledge in both older people and staff, and how this conspires against keeping them warm at home. In conclusion, the relevance of these findings on some aspects of policy and practice is reflected upon.

The research and its findings

Full details of the methods used in KWILLT can be accessed elsewhere (Tod et al. 2012). In brief, semi-structured in-depth interviews were conducted with 50 older people. Interviews were conducted after seven days of hourly temperature measurements were recorded. Measurements were taken in the rooms in which they spent most of the day and night. Older participants were recruited via health and social care staff who worked with older people in their home, as well as community and faith groups and community workers. Purposive and snowball sampling was used to ensure the sample included socially isolated older people.

In addition, 25 health and social care staff who worked with older people were recruited to participate in semi-structured individual interviews. Participants included practice and district nurses, community physiotherapists and occupational therapists, domiciliary care workers, community wardens, debt advisors, housing advisers and general practitioners. Findings from the individual interviews were tested further and expanded upon in six focus groups conducted with a total of 43 participants. There were three groups with older people, one with staff, and two with strategic leads in the public and third sector. Framework analysis methods were used to develop a thematic framework, code and interpret the data (Ritchie and Lewis 2003; Tod et al. 2012).

The findings from the study were used to develop six pen portraits (Tod et al. 2012). These are not real people, but case studies that describe how the complex network of interrelated factors come together in six groups of older people to place them at risk of being cold at home. Whilst the findings here focus on information and knowledge deficits, it may be useful to look at the pen portraits to understand how these issues play out alongside other themes and barriers identified (http://www.kwillt.org).

Older people

The older people who participated in the study had deficits in information and knowledge related to the link between warmth and health, safe room temperatures and technology (heating, computers and finance). Illustrative examples of each of these now follow.

Warmth and health: legacies from the past

Overall, our participants did not understand that being warm had a protective impact on health and being cold could be harmful. Most described past experiences of hardship and hardiness where homes were poorly heated. Most grew up in solid fuel heated homes where only those rooms with a fire were warm, or the amount of fuel used would depend on when the next coal delivery was due or could be afforded. Bedrooms were rarely heated in their younger years. Some thought that warm rooms (especially bedrooms) were harmful or an unnecessary luxury.

> They probably see heating as a luxury as well because when they were younger they didn't have heated houses did they? They had a coal fire and that would heat just one room.
>
> *(Staff interviewee; Community health professional)*

> [being] too warm, that's unhealthy isn't it?
>
> *(Older person participant, female, 76 years)*

Safe room temperatures

No participants were aware that there was a recommended 'safe' temperature for the home (Department of Health 2012a, 2012b; Marmot Review Team 2011),[2] or that people should keep all the rooms in use at a safe temperature over the day. In the past people were advised to heat the room they were in to cut down on cost. However, physiological stress can result from moving from a warm room to cold areas in the house and there is an increased risk of falling.

> They get to the stage where they will switch it off, they'll wrap up but they don't understand the importance of the house being warm because they've lived in conditions like that for many years when they were younger, damp cold houses, and they don't realise the effect it can have on their health.
>
> *(Staff interviewee; Domiciliary Care Manager)*

Older participants did not believe it was more fuel efficient to keep the heating on and across the home. They preferred to adopt other strategies rather than warming the house. For example they would 'layer up' with extra clothes, blankets and hot water bottles. In general a warm bedroom was considered unhealthy.

Boilers, timers and the internet

Vulnerability to cold for some was exacerbated by technology. Participants described how they struggled to 'work' their heating. Most had lived in solid fuel housing for the majority of their life and now struggled with understanding how their central heating boiler worked, how to set the programmer and what a thermostat was for. There were practical as well as information barriers as age and infirmity made it harder to reach awkwardly placed boilers and programmers, turn knobs or see programming dials and clocks.

> Sometimes I feel quite cold, and I don't know why that is. I don't know how to work that one in there. That's why I just said to him, when he set it for me, I said look I want to work it manually. I want it going off and coming on when I want to do it. So I just work from the thermostat in the hall and just come down in the morning, switch it on, and when I go up at night I switch it off. You know, so I don't know the first thing about working that boiler.
>
> *(Older person participant, female, 71 years)*

A recurrent theme was struggling with the internet. Previously, people would have seen leaflets or posters but now much material is electronic, including the UK national Keep Warm, Keep Well campaign (DH 2012c). Whilst some embraced innovation, others did not want, like or understand the technology. This heightened feelings of social isolation and disconnection. It also meant that people did not access cheaper, online fuel tariffs or payment methods, such as direct debits. People preferred older processes such as paying for utilities by cheque or cash and getting a paper bill and receipt. The invisibility of electronic and online finance transactions were confusing and bewildering to some.

> I don't think they know how to set the timers and things. A lady I went to, hers was on the stairs and she didn't have a clue. She just put the boiler on every day and that was it. And her house was quite cold because she only had it on for certain times of the day but she did have an electric heater which she plugged in which was at the side of her to keep her warm. She wasn't really bothered about the rest of the house. They keep themselves warm, they sit with blankets on. But I don't think they know how to work these new systems. I don't actually, I leave it to my husband.
>
> *(Staff interviewee; Community health professional)*

> They'll not do direct debits a lot of them, they don't know how to do it . . . even writing a cheque basically, almost impossible for a lot of older people because they don't know, they've never done it; they've always dealt in cash.
>
> *(Staff participant; Financial Inclusion Advisor)*

This lack of knowledge created situations where people did not recognise they were at risk or needed help and so struggled on by themselves. Attitudes and values sometimes prevented people accessing help; for example, stoicism, valuing hardiness and thrift, protecting privacy and independence, liking routine and disliking change. However, there was a widespread mistrust of key organisations who could help. Key examples here included local government, banks and energy companies. Media coverage exacerbated existing mistrust of such organisations, meaning people often did not access the cheaper tariffs. The cumulative effect of these influences was that older people found it impossible to navigate their way through the number of organisations and fragmented systems to access help.

Staff knowledge and assumptions

The staff who were interviewed also described how deficiencies in their knowledge and awareness may mean those at risk of being cold at home are unidentified or do not get referred for help. They reported lack of knowledge related to the health risks of a cold home, what safe temperatures were, what could be done to help people and by whom.

> I don't think people actually associate heat, warmth with health at all. I mean I have to say, as a health visitor and a nurse, for goodness knows how many years, it's only when affordable warmth became sort of being promoted that I really linked the two. So, you know, even as a health professional I haven't really given it a great deal of thought.
>
> *(Staff interviewee; public health specialist)*

This is explained and illustrated further here by relating a number of assumptions people expressed on their own behalf or those of their colleagues:

- *People aren't cold these days*: staff described scenarios of overheating being more problematic than underheating. However, rates of EWDs and increased winter hospital admissions bear testament to risk for some older people because of cold. There are physiological reasons why some older people are unable to maintain their body temperature in a room that is suitably warm for a younger, active person (Worfolk 1997). It is perfectly possible that busy health staff may dash in to see an older person and not be aware the room is cold enough to be a health risk.
- *It's only the really old who are affected*: staff assumed that it was only the really old and infirm who were at risk of being cold at home. In KWILLT some of our younger participants were the most at risk due to chronic co-morbidity, for example, mental health and cardiovascular disease, and poor environment and housing.
- *Only people who are fuel poor are cold*: the findings clearly illustrate how attitudes and values may place some older people who are not fuel poor at risk of being cold.
- *Family will tackle the problems*: there was an assumption that if older patients and clients had family members living close by they would make sure the older person was warm. In KWILLT some family members also lacked the knowledge and awareness to help vulnerable relatives.

- *People know what healthy temperatures are and that there are health impacts of being cold*: some staff participants indicated that people knew that being cold was bad for you and that is was an informed choice not to heat the home. There was sometimes a reluctance to interfere or challenge people's heating practices.
- *People know how to use technology:* staff exhibited a lack of awareness of the barriers some older people encounter in terms of understanding how to use the heating and how to get the most preferential tariff. In fact, staff described similar challenges themselves.
- *Vulnerable people read and act on health and energy efficiency information:* staff participants did not understand that some people make heating decisions based on past experience and values built up over years, rather than on an information campaign from a mistrusted source.
- *Someone else will deal with it:* some staff participants were unaware of who can help if someone was cold at home, or they assumed someone else would intervene. Others struggled to find the right person or organisation to help.

The above findings indicate how older people and staff can end up without the information and resources to promote healthy temperatures and heating behaviour in those vulnerable to negative health impacts of cold weather. Some of the implications of these findings for policy and practice will now be explored.

Application to policy and practice

The methods adopted in KWILLT provided a unique insight into the decision making and behaviour of older people in relation to home heating. KWILLT has provided understanding of the complex home environment and highlights the need for organisations to work in partnership in identifying, assessing, referring and delivering help to those who need it. The study reinforces findings from others that the public and staff lack awareness of the health risks of cold and that people are reluctant to ask for help in case they were seen to be struggling (Critchley et al. 2007; Day and Hitchings 2011; Hitchings and Day 2011; Wright 2004).

The findings raise some public health challenges. They indicate fuel poverty can be overlaid by other issues such as a lack of awareness, information and knowledge. This means vulnerable older people struggle to operate in their own environment, have control over their lives or live in a healthy and sustainable place.

Identifying people at risk is crucial (Department of Health 2012a) and the six KWILLT pen portraits mentioned earlier can assist (see Figure 17.1 and the project website http:// kwillt.org/). The pen portraits can help relevant organisations and individuals to find and recognise people who are at risk and understand the complex reasons why older people are cold. In this way organisations can design and deliver acceptable and accessible interventions to overcome barriers and promote strategies to support self-management to keep warm. The pen portraits have been used to develop education and training DVDs, e-learning materials and the Winter Warmth England website.[3]

Even if staff awareness and skills in assessment of the vulnerable are improved little

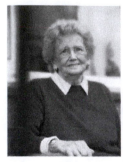

Lonely, Pearle

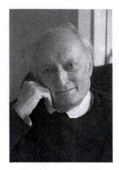

Proud, Fred

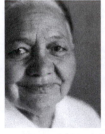

Dependent, Meena

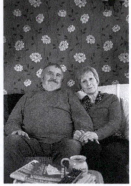

Getting by, Bob and Joan

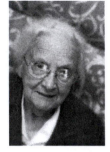

Just about managing, Enid

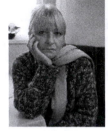

Isolated, Pat

FIGURE 17.1 KWILLT pen portraits.

will change unless pathways to help are available. In order to achieve this, partnership schemes are required. Those likely to be successful and accessible to the vulnerable are those that operate a single point of contact. The issues raised in KWILLT illustrate how bewildering it can be for an older vulnerable person to navigate systems and access help.

Building individual and community resilience and competency is challenging, especially for those who are socially isolated, old and/or frail. Helping people to recognise and deal with cold as a health risk may require resource and input from someone people already have a trusting relationship with. Community and primary care health staff or domiciliary care providers may therefore be well placed to initiate a conversation and begin the process of promoting heating behaviour change. Whilst it is not appropriate for care staff to be experts in energy efficiency, what is useful is if they are aware of risk, able to conduct an initial assessment of risk and refer accordingly. At the time of writing there is concern that NHS and local authority organisations will be less well resourced to embrace this role, as they struggle with financial and staffing constraints. This creates even more urgency for multi-sector partnerships with voluntary and community organisations, lay initiatives such as health champions as well as energy efficiency schemes run by energy providers.[4]

Conclusion

The factors that place older people at risk of the negative health impacts of cold weather are varied, complex and interactional. Qualitative approaches are required to understand how different factors play out in the context of people's lives. There is a need for concerted effort to raise public and staff awareness of the risk and improve ability to identify the vulnerable. Creative solutions are required to build, maintain and resource partnership systems and pathways to help and support. The methods used in KWILLT proved effective in capturing and disseminating the lay voice in a way that can be used to challenge traditional ways of understanding health risk. The methods supported the development of applied resources that organisations can use to help them plan and respond to that need. Such methods have great potential for use in other public health areas.

Notes

1   The study was independent research commissioned by the National Institute for Health Research (NIHR) under its Research for Patient Benefit (RfPB) Programme (Grant Reference Number PB-PG-0408-16041) and supported by the Collaboration for Leadership in Applied Health Research and Care (CLAHRC) South Yorkshire. The views expressed are those of the authors and not necessarily those of the NHS, the NIHR or the Department of Health.
2   Most health advice in the UK adopts World Health Organisation recommendations for safe room temperatures. These are 21° in the room during the day and 18° in the bedroom at night.
3   KWILLT materials are available on the project website (http://kwillt.org/) and Winter Warmth England Website (http://www.winterwarmthengland.co.uk/).
4   Community Health Champions are people who, with training and support, work voluntarily with families, communities and workplaces to promote health, facilitate involvement in healthy social activities, create groups to meet local needs and signpost people to relevant support and services.

References

Allmark, P. and Tod, A. M. (2006) How should public health professionals engage with lay epidemiology? *Journal of Medical Ethics* 32: 460–463.

Critchley, R., Gilbertson, J., Grimsley, M. and Green, G. and the Warm Front Study Group (2007) Living in cold homes after heating improvements: evidence from Warm Front, England's Home Energy Efficiency Scheme. *Applied Energy* 84: 147–158.

Davison, C., Frankel, S. and Smith, G. D. (1992) The limits of life-style: reassessing fatalism in the popular culture of illness prevention. *Social Science and Medicine* 34: 675–685.

Davison, C., Smith, G. D. and Frankel, S. (1991) Lay epidemiology and the prevention paradox: the implications of coronary candidacy for health-education. *Sociology of Health and Illness* 13: 1–19.

Day, R. and Hitchings, R. (2011) 'Only old ladies would do that': age stigma and older people's strategies for dealing with winter cold. *Health and Place* 17, 4: 885–894. doi:10.1016/j.healthplace.2011.04.011.

Department of Health (2011) *Cold Weather Plan for England: Making the Case: Why Cold Weather Planning Is Essential to Health and Wellbeing.* London: Department of Health.

Department of Health (2012a) *Cold Weather Plan for England: Protecting Health and Reducing Harm from Severe Cold.* London: Department of Health.

Department of Health (2012b) *Cold Weather Plan for England: Supporting the Case*. London: Department of Health.

Department of Health (2012c) *Keep Warm Keep Well*. Online at: http://www.nhs.uk/Livewell/winterhealth/Documents/KeepWarmKeepWell2012.pdf Accessed July 2013.

Department of Health (2013) Public Health Outcomes Framework (PHOF) 2013–2016. Online at: https://www.gov.uk/government/publications/healthy-lives-healthy-people-improving-outcomes-and-supporting-transparency Accessed December 2013.

Frankel, S., Davison, C. and Smith, G. D. (1991) Lay epidemiology and the rationality of responses to health-education. *British Journal of General Practice* 41: 428–430.

Health and Social Care Act 2012. Online at: http://www.legislation.gov.uk/ukpga/2012/7/contents/enacted Accessed September 2013.

Hitchings, R. and Day, R. (2011) How older people relate to the private winter warmth practices of their peers and why we should be interested. *Environment and Planning* 43: 2452–2467.

Marmot Review (2010) *Fair Society, Healthy Lives*. London: The Marmot Review.

Marmot Review Team (2011) *The Health Impacts of Cold Homes and Fuel Poverty*. London: Friends of the Earth.

Office of National Statistics (2012) *Excess Winter Mortality in England and Wales, 2011/12 (Provisional) and 2010/11 (Final)*. Online at: http://www.ons.gov.uk/ons/rel/subnational-health2/excess-winter-mortality-in-england-and-wales/2011-12--provisional--and-2010-11--final-/index.html Accessed September 2013.

Ritchie, J. and Lewis, J. (2003) *Qualitative Research Practice: A Guide for Social Science Students and Researchers*. London: Sage.

Tod, A. M., Lusambili, A., Homer, C., Abbott, J., Cooke, J. M., Stocks, A. J. and McDaid, K. A. (2012) Understanding factors influencing vulnerable older people keeping warm and well in winter: a qualitative study using social marketing techniques. *BMJ Open* 2, 4. doi:10.1136/bmjopen-2012-000922.

Worfolk, J. B. (1997) Keep frail elders warm! *Geriatric Nursing* 18, 1: 7–11.

Wright, F. (2004) Old and cold: older people and policies failing to address fuel poverty. *Social Policy and Administration* 38, 5: 488–503.

18

CONCLUSION

Looking to the future

Angela M. Tod, Julia Hirst and Peter Allmark

Introduction

This concluding chapter is a reflection on the future of public health; it pulls together some key themes and points of learning raised in the previous chapters. This is achieved, first, in relation to two landmark reports, The Black Report, entitled *Inequalities in Health* (DHSS 1980), and *Fair Society, Healthy Lives* (Marmot Review 2010). Second, the chapter considers some of the challenges, priorities and opportunities for public health in forthcoming years. The chapter will include reference to implications for research for public health.

As with the rest of this book, cognisance of the role of wider social determinants on health and the influence of the broader political landscape will be at the forefront of the deliberations (Dahlgren and Whitehead 1991). Whilst the book and this chapter focus on the United Kingdom (UK) many of the reflections, lessons and challenges can be applied to other International contexts. Issues of social injustice, political change and economic turbulence will have an impact on public health across the world. Whilst the detail of experiences may vary according to the histories, cultures and infrastructures of specific nations, it is possible to identify key messages that apply to all.

Public health – reflections on inequalities and Marmot

The Health Divide – a call for action

Our book took as its starting point the Black Report (DHSS 1980). This ground-breaking report revealed that, despite the improvements in overall health since the introduction of the welfare state and NHS, those from lower occupational groups in Britain still experienced worse health, and that this economic inequality accounted for the class gradient in mortality. Importantly, Black, and subsequently Whitehead (1987) and Townsend et al. (1990), demonstrated that many of the factors contributing to this gradient and inequality lay outside of the NHS and in the broader realms of public health.

'Social and economic factors like income, work (or lack of it), environment, education, housing, transport and what are today called 'lifestyles' all affect health and all favour the better off.' (Townsend et al. 1990: 2).

The Black Report is widely recognised as a pioneering text and set the agenda for public health for the next 30 years. In this sense, it was a call for action. The suggestion was that without something being done at a political level, health inequalities would only get worse. Redressing the balance and improving the material conditions of life for those experiencing inequalities were at the heart of public health responses to the challenges in the Black Report and *The Health Divide* (Townsend et al. 1990). Later public health policy and interventions echoed the debate that followed *The Health Divide*, such as the establishment of Health Action Zones by the 1997 Labour government. Whilst of limited success, Health Action Zones (HAZ) were based in geographical areas of inequality and emphasised the role of partnership working (health, local government, voluntary sector and private industry) to overcome some of the material and economic disadvantage at the root of health inequalities. In effect, HAZ policy acknowledged the controversy between individual and state accountability and responsibility for health. Another initiative was the development of the Health Inequalities National Support Team, whose work and frameworks for action are considered in Chapter 2.

Marmot – a map for the future?

It is proposed in Chapters 1 and 2 of this book that the UK Marmot Report *Fair Society, Healthy Lives* (Marmot Review 2010) provides a mark in the sand for public health today, as much as the Black Report did in its day. Marmot maps out the scope of the current challenge and provides a waymark for public health in the future. In his initial international report conducted for the World Health Organisation, *Closing the Gap in a Generation* (Commission on the Social Determinants of Health 2008), Marmot focuses on the need to address existing social injustices, the poor material conditions people work and live in, and the need to expand the evidence base to facilitate better social awareness and effective public health action. These tenets are fundamental to *Fair Society, Healthy Lives*. In some ways it picks up the mantle laid down by Townsend, Davidson and Whitehead (1990) to acknowledge the size and complexity of health inequalities in the UK and recognise the need for an evidence base that reflects the enormity and intricacy of the task ahead. It does this by stating clear public health policy goals and objectives throughout the lifespan. It is the lifespan stages within *Fair Society, Healthy Lives* (2010) that form the structure of the work presented in this book.

However, in Chapter 2, Bentley considers some aspects of the *Fair Society, Healthy Lives* report that provide challenges for the future. Key points made by Bentley are summarised below. Whilst these points are made in relation to the UK, they could apply to other international contexts.

- In order to make a difference to health inequalities on any scale, impact needs to be made at a population level. However, the report lacks detail and remains vague in that it does not provide principles for driving population-level change. There is a call to action, but a lack of detail in terms of the plan of action. This can impede implementation and achievement of the policy objectives.

- Many of the recommendations on delivery within the Marmot Report are addressed as structures and processes that were present at the time of writing, for example, Primary Care Trusts, NHS Regional Offices, Local Strategic Partnerships. However, as is typical with public health in many countries, political change, such as a change of government administration, can mean that the environment where public health policy is implemented is very different to that in which it was commissioned. Such was the case here. The UK Government elected in 2010 instituted radical programmes of reform and restructuring including the movement of public health departments from the NHS to local authorities. It can be argued that in the long term this could be an advantage as many of the wider social determinants of health can be seen to be the business of local authorities, such as environment, adult and child services, neighbourhoods and education. However, in the short term there has been a period of relative inactivity whilst new structures have been established and organisational change implemented. This illustrates a fundamental challenge for public health, that is, how to function to maximum population impact whilst continually adapting to external political change?

- Bentley (Chapter 2) takes issue with a principle of 'proportionate universalism' (Marmot Review 2010: 16). The principle suggests that if the gradient of inequality in life expectancy is to be substantially reduced, action will be required across the whole spectrum. Whilst this is true, Bentley argues that in addition, families and individuals who experience multiple disadvantages require *disproportionate* inputs to make the same gains as for people in other parts of the 'gradient'. The importance of this is not fully acknowledged in the Marmot reports.

- The contribution of individual practitioners to individual lives must be applauded and facilitated in terms of addressing health inequalities. However, changes are required at a population level to address fundamental social injustices and the material conditions of those in need. Again, detail is lacking in Marmot to inform such activity. As Bentley highlights:

  > Translating such ideals into practice in the real world will require interventions with the power to bring about 'sea-change' in circumstances and outcomes. What are the characteristics of such interventions and to what extent can policy proposals be translated into delivery systems capable of producing percentage change at population level?

- Bentley argues that population change requires interventions that are multi-layered, at population, service and community level. Community-level intervention needs to be based on genuine and effective community engagement, collaboration and accurate insight.

- Finally and importantly, Bentley draws attention to the 'decay model'. Drawn from evidence in relation to medical interventions, the model illustrates how those most in need of an intervention may find it inaccessible. Various reasons may account for this, including personal capacity, organisational effectiveness or service quality. In public health there is a requirement to ensure that the interventions that aim to address inequalities do not exacerbate them. This can occur when an intervention is impossible to access for those most in need but easier for those less vulnerable to a health threat. For example, to what extent do strategies to increase uptake of screening speed up access to those who would be screened anyway, rather than increase uptake of those most at risk? Health inequality interventions require evidence rooted in user insight and should avoid a one-size-fits-all approach.

Having considered some of the key challenges to public health that can be drawn from a critique of the Marmot Review (2010), attention now turns to a few main messages emerging from the public health research and evaluation projects presented in the book.

Public health messages for the future

Taking *Fair Society, Healthy Lives* (Marmot Review 2010) as a structure, this book presents two public health research or evaluation projects at each point of the lifespan. Each project illustrates aspects of health inequalities, provides unique insight into factors that contribute to these and proposes possible strategies and implications for public health practice and policy. The topics covered are diverse and the methods used varied. However, by reflecting on the overall content of the book it is possible to identify some key, simple messages that are pertinent for evidence based public health in the future. Three of these are considered below.

1 Evidence not assumption

Underpinning both the Black and Marmot Reports is an acceptance of a social gradient of inequalities. Added to this, as mentioned above, is the notion that families, individuals and communities subject to multiple disadvantages require *disproportionate* inputs to make the same gains as for people in other parts of the 'gradient'. Public health strategies and interventions are required that address these inequalities, whether by shifting the whole gradient up or investing in those at disproportionate advantage. If these interventions are to be effective it is essential that public health measures are informed by an understanding of how wider determinants of health operate from the perspective of those experiencing adversity. In this way public health policy and interventions will be grounded in evidence, and in the experiences of the vulnerable. Public health should not be rooted in the assumptions and beliefs of politicians, professionals and influential partisan stakeholders, for example the tobacco or food industry. By examining the content of the work presented in the previous chapters it is possible to see how assumptions of health professionals may mean health services remain difficult to access for people (see Poll, Chapter 11 on people with hepatitis C). Similarly, public health policy based on false assumptions can mean vulnerable older people remain cold because they are unable to use technology to access cheaper fuel tariffs or respond to interventions in a way fuel companies or housing organisations expect (see Tod, Chapter 17). In some cases, public health assumptions are derived from sound epidemiological data, such as those linking smoking to lung cancer which inform stop smoking campaigns. However, it is necessary to understand 'lay epidemiology' alongside 'traditional epidemiology'. Lay epidemiology refers to the network of attitudes, values and knowledge that people build up over their life that influences their behaviour and comes from many varied, trusted sources. Without basing public health interventions on an understanding of lay epidemiology, there is a risk they will be assumption- rather than evidence-based. Public response may be very different to that anticipated by public health experts (Allmark and Tod 2006).

Just like any health intervention, public health interventions can have negative consequences and unwanted side effects. Examples include public health information campaigns that seek to promote one action, e.g. stopping smoking, but inadvertently contribute to unanticipated behaviour, e.g. delay in reporting emerging symptoms of lung cancer leading to a delay in diagnosis (Allmark and Tod 2009; Allmark et al. 2007). It is therefore important to ensure that public health interventions undergo the same level of evaluation and scrutiny to understand the nature of their impact as does any other health intervention, such as a drug–based response.

The messages are therefore to challenge assumption-based practice and policy and seek out evidence and insight to understand public health risk and vulnerability.

2 Complexity, change and multi-layered responses

Further challenges to public health lie in the increasing complexity and continual change of the environment within which it works. Nationally, in 2013, a raft of new UK policy and legislation was introduced in areas impacting upon public health including health, energy, housing, welfare, education and local government. Alongside this was an economic recession that created new and exacerbated existing inequalities (Ramesh 2013). Internationally, new public health dilemmas and challenges emerge in response to volatile political situations, for example, civil unrest and uprising in Egypt and Syria and in the Middle East. In parallel there is rapid and fundamental global economic change. At the time of writing, Western, developed countries like the UK have experienced an economic downturn, whilst other economies, such as China and India, are strengthening on the back of new mineral development, new markets and large workforce. The size and nature of this change means it is difficult to grasp where power and vulnerability lie in terms of public health, whether in relation to refugee communities from war torn nations or deprived communities in areas where previous heavy industry is now redundant. It is testing to develop effective and sustainable public health strategies in such an environment. However, a key message to emerge from this book is that it is important to look for knowledge and solutions at a population, community and individual (micro) level. Multi-layered responses are required for complex problems. It is not sufficient to focus only on the behaviour of an individual without looking at the political, economic and cultural drivers, influences and constraints that influence it. Finally, in the context of the complexity and change discussed here it is necessary to consider who the public health workforce will be in the future. In the UK it is an interesting time to ask. Those who work as public health professionals have found themselves uprooted from a medically dominated NHS setting to a socially and politically driven local government setting. This potentially changes who sits round the public health table at a local level and should help collaborative public health endeavour between local government departments. However, such is the extent of the challenge in public health today that it would serve us well to broaden our ideas of *who* has a role to play in promoting and protecting health and wellbeing, and *what* those roles are. In the work displayed in these chapters we see a vast array of staff and lay people making a valuable contribution to public health achievements. These include childminders, prison officers, drug workers, energy companies, welfare advice officers, housing officers, school teachers, as well as volunteers working as advisors, role models, peer support, health trainers and counsellors. For a more detailed discussion of the role of the public, and lay roles in public health and community engagement see the work of South et al. (2011, 2012, 2013). It is necessary to embrace and value the contribution of everyone to achieve positive health outcomes and address inequalities, irrespective of status, profession, economic standing and social and cultural capital.

3 Individual versus state accountability

Underpinning much public health debate prior to and including the Black Report is the notion of where responsibility and accountability lie for public health action, and health protection and promotion. Opinion in this debate is often polarised with participants adopting their position in line with their various political, ideological or economic positions. On one side, libertarians oppose government policy interventions that can threaten individual rights and control. Allegations of 'nanny-state' and government paternalism are made in response to legislative and population-based measures such as regulation of marketing or advertising of unhealthy products such as tobacco or sugary drinks (Wiley et al. 2013). Those who contest what they view as 'nanny-state' government interference affiliate to lifestyle approaches that hold individuals morally and financially responsible for their health choices and behaviour. No or little credence is placed upon theories of wider determinants that contribute to vulnerability, constrain choice or sense of control.

On the opposing side are those who propose society as partly responsible for the health of its citizens, access to health supporting environments are a social responsibility, with the state having accountability to maintain the promotion and protection of health (Resnick 2007). This side of the lobby also support upstream approaches to health and illness prevention, rather than focusing on downstream health care delivery and treatment (McKinlay 1975; Resnick 2007). This debate has been played out with regard to various public health priorities in the past such as water fluoridation, seatbelt and motorcycle helmet laws and tobacco. More recently the arguments are sharpened and delivered in relation to measures to address obesity. Individual choice, rights and responsibility are cited by libertarians on one side, with regulation on the other, for example, limiting portion sizes, calorific value of foods and advertising (see Feinberg 1984 and Skrabanek 1990 for libertarian perspectives).

Such polarity is not necessarily helpful. In recent years, two contributions to the debate have provided a way forward and are helpful to consider in the public health of the future. First, in 2007 the Nuffield Council on Bioethics (Nuffield 2007) published its report on public health ethical issues. Produced by a working party of experts in ethics, law and evidence-based healthcare, the report recognised the debate above, sought a way forward and considered the responsibilities of government, industry and individuals. The Report proposes a 'Stewardship Model' that delicately balances the responsibilities of the state and individuals. It lists public health policy goals that address health risks external to individuals, environmental conditions, vulnerabilities of certain populations and issues of access and equity. On the other hand, it states policy should not be coercive, be implemented without consultation and evidence, or be intrusive to individuals (Nuffield 2007). In addition, an 'Intervention Ladder' is proposed to guide public health policy makers in establishing that the level of intervention (interference) is proportionate to the level and likelihood of anticipated benefit. The ladder helps to assess how interventions may limit individuals' choices; the higher the level of the intervention, the greater the limitation on choice and, therefore, the stronger the justification that is required. For example, legislation to require seat-belt wearing forcibly restricts choice; however, the choice is not perceived important by many and the health payoff is great. Finally, Nuffield highlights that, not only the state but also industry and business have a social responsibility for the health effect of those products. When industry does not behave responsibly it is acceptable for the state to intervene. The Stewardship Model and Intervention Ladder provide useful tools for reflection and guidance for people working at all levels of public health.

The second response to the polarised debate regarding state versus individual comes from Wiley et al. (2013). They recommend reframing the debate in order to move forward to a more productive position. The 'nanny-state' position is a distraction that moves attention away from public health and towards 'government overreach' (Wiley et al. 2012: 88). This tactic protects the interests of those who may not be well served by legislation or regulation, such as sugary food manufacturers and advertisers. Instead it is proposed that the 'nanny-state' framing is replaced by a more positive 'vision of community action', replacing notions of lifestyle interventions and individual responsibility with those of democratic process and collective problem solving (Wiley et al. 2013: 90). This focuses attention back to the community-based responses and activity described by Bentley in Chapter 2, and refocuses debate towards collective approaches to building healthier communities (Wiley et al. 2013: 90).

Having briefly discussed some complex concepts and ideas that emerge from the current debates in public health, and the content of this book, the implications for public health research are now considered.

Messages for public health research

As demonstrated previously, public health works in a complex changing world, politically, ideologically and academically. World economies and governments change, and new, different and nuanced ideological and academic positions are adopted by governing bodies. Public health is tasked to keep pace with this change. In doing so, it needs to develop its intelligence and evidence base to effectively inform the core function of promoting and protecting health and wellbeing.

Though 20 years old, the proposals in the Leeds Declaration (Long 1993) still hold true (see Chapter 1). The public health challenges and research projects presented in this book illustrate the value of the Declaration. For example, focusing upstream to the worlds of work and welfare helps us understand the social structures and processes within which ill-health originates. The in-depth inquiry of Hirst, Formby and Tod (Chapters 7, 8 and 17) show how research can generate knowledge of the subtle ways that complex, interrelated factors keep some people healthy and others ill. Common throughout the book is a recognition of the value of lay knowledge and how harnessing people's experience can teach us about health needs, health service priorities and health outcomes. In order to achieve this insight in public health a plurality of research methods is required (see Albertson et al., Chapter 5). The important message is to choose the right tool, or mix of tools, for the job. As Long claims:

> There is nothing inherently 'soft' about qualitative methods or 'hard' about quantitative methods – both require rigorous application in appropriate contexts and hard thinking about difficult problems.
>
> *(Long 1994: 253)*

The public health evaluation and research presented in this book provide sound examples of the contribution of qualitative methods to public health inquiry. Many of the projects are small, interview-based studies. Whilst caution is required in claiming transferability and generalisability of qualitative data, its advantages should not be underplayed. Qualitative approaches provide a mechanism to capture the experience and voices of those who may find it impossible to engage with more traditional, experimental research, even if such approaches are appropriate to answering some public health questions, such as those that expose changes and trends over the longer term. For some people research participation in an experimental study may be impossible or difficult due to a perceived or real burden. Taking part in an interview may be an acceptable, or the only, way to capture those people's voices and experiences. Examples here include those with severe, chronic mental health problems (see Pollard, Chapter 16), the socially isolated (see Tod, Chapter 17), and those experiencing shame, blame and stigma (Formby, Reece and Clack, and Poll, Chapters 8, 10 and 11). Without such qualitative approaches there is a risk that public health policy and interventions will be informed by research that excludes those most at risk.

In brief, in relation to public health research and evidence, our final question is what can be learnt from the knowledge and experience derived from the research, evaluation and discussion within this book?

- The proposals laid down in the Leeds Declaration are still appropriate today. They serve as a template for reflection when reading, assessing, applying and generating public health evidence for the future.

- It is not justified to base public health policy and interventions on assumptions about how people will behave, even if these assumptions are derived from epidemiological data. Robust research is required to develop in-depth evidence to understand how people navigate their everyday world and how vulnerability is experienced in relation to health. Without such insight public health measures may fall on fallow ground, or more importantly may have negative, unwanted consequences. This point is similar to that made by Pawson in relation to realist evaluation (Pawson and Tilley 1997; Pawson et al. 2005). A particular intervention might lead to a particular outcome but the mechanism by which it does so is important. He gives an example. Money given to prisoners as they leave prison might reduce recidivism over a year. But the mechanism could be (a) it gives them space to find legitimate work or (b) it makes it unnecessary to commit crime for a bit. Whilst epidemiological research has shown that the measure works in reducing crime, the lack of qualitative data to show how it works will almost certainly portend failure when the measure is rolled out.
- As the public health world becomes more complex and rapidly changing, research and evaluation methods need to develop and evolve accordingly. New and creative approaches are required, along with new combinations and mixtures of methods. Community-based research, using innovative sampling strategies and data collection techniques, will be needed more than ever. The public health research world of the future will demand new collaborative approaches across public, private and voluntary sectors, academic disciplines, economic environments and international boundaries. The voice of the lay person and their everyday world must be central to this.

Conclusion

In this book we have reflected on key public health policy to establish a context within which to examine some public health policy and practice challenges. A range of research and evaluation projects have been summarised to illustrate some of the diverse approaches to understanding public health and generating insight to inform future practice. Lessons and reflections have been drawn from this content. Public health has probably never faced such a complex range of challenges. However, this book provides some strategies to increase the reflexivity of policy makers, practitioners and researchers. It also demonstrates the value of collaboration and the necessity to adopt multi-layered approaches to public health problems and evaluation.

References

Allmark, P. and Tod, A. M. (2006) How should public health professionals engage with lay epidemiology? *Journal of Medical Ethics* 32: 460–463.

Allmark, P. and Tod, A. M. (2009) The evaluation of public health education initiatives on smoking and lung cancer: an ethical critique. In S. Peckham and A. Hann (eds) *Public Health Ethics and Practice*. London: Policy Press, Chapter 5, pp. 65–81.

Allmark, P., Tod, A. M. and Abbott, J. (2007) Philosophy and health education: the case of lung cancer and smoking. In J. Drummond and P. Standish (eds) *The Philosophy of Nurse Education*. London: Palgrave Macmillan.

Black, D. (1982) *Inequalities in Health: Black Report.* London: Penguin Books.

Commission on the Social Determinants of Health (2008) *Closing the Gap in a Generation.* Geneva: World Health Organisation.

Dahlgren, G. and Whitehead, M. (1991) *Policies and Strategies to Promote Social Equity in Health.* Stockholm, Sweden: Institute for Futures Studies.

DHSS (1980) *The Black Report: Inequalities in Health: Report of a Research Working Group.* London: DHSS. Online at: http://www.sochealth.co.uk/public-health-and-wellbeing/poverty-and-inequality/the-black-report-1980/ Accessed September 2013.

Feinberg J. (1984) *Harm to Others: The Moral Limits of the Criminal Law.* New York: Oxford University Press.

Long, A. F. (1993) *Understanding Health and Disease: Towards a Knowledge Base for Public Health Action.* Report of Workshop. Leeds: Nuffield Institute for Health.

Long, A. F. (1994) Directions for health: new approaches to population health research and practice – the Leeds Declaration. *Journal of Public Health* 16, 3: 253–255.

Long, A. F. (1997) The Leeds Declaration: three years on – a symbol or a catalyst for change? *Critical Public Health* 7, 1–2: 73–81. Online at: http://dx.doi.org/10.1080/09581599708409080.

McKinlay, J. B. (1975) A case for refocusing upstream: the political economy of sickness. In A. J. Enelow and J. B. Henderson (eds) *Applying Behavioral Science to Cardiovascular Risk.* Washington, DC: American Heart Association.

Marmot Review (2010) *Fair Society, Healthy Lives.* Online at: http://www.instituteofhealthequity.org/projects/fair-society-healthy-lives-the-marmot-review/fair-society-healthy-lives-full-report Accessed September 2013.

Nuffield Council on Bioethics (2007) Public Health Ethical Issues. Online at: http://www.nuffieldbioethics.org/public-health#3 Accessed September 2013.

Ramesh, R. (2013) Young and poor hit hardest as UK cuts widen inequality, says OECD. *Guardian,* 15 May 2013. Online at: http://www.theguardian.com/society/2013/may/15/cuts-inequality-oecd Accessed September 2013.

Resnick, D. (2007) Responsibility for health: personal, social and environmental. *Journal of Medical Ethics* 33: 444–445.

Skrabanek, P. (1990) Why is preventive medicine exempted from ethical constraints? *Journal of Medical Ethics* 16: 187–190 doi:10.1136/jme.16.4.18.

South, J., Jackson, K. L. and Warwick-Booth, L. (2011) The community health apprentices project: the outcomes of an intermediate labour market project in the community health sector. *Community, Work and Family* 14, 1: 1–18.

South, J., Meah, A. and Branney, P. (2012) 'Think differently and be prepared to demonstrate trust': findings from public hearings, England, on supporting lay people in public health roles. *Health Promotion International* 27, 2 (June): 284–294.

South, J., White, J., Branney, P. and Kinsella, K. (2013) Public health skills for a lay workforce: findings on skills and attributes from a qualitative study of lay health worker roles. *Public Health* 127, 5 (May): 419–426.

Townsend, P., Davidson, N. and Whitehead, M. (1990) *Inequalities in Health: The Black Report and The Health Divide.* London: Penguin.

Whitehead, M. (1987) *The Health Divide: Inequalities in Health.* London: Health Education Council, UK.

Wiley, L., Berman, M. and Blanke, D. (2013) Who's your nanny? Choice, paternalism and public health in the age of personal responsibility. *Journal of Law, Medicine and Ethics* 41 (s1): 88–91.

INDEX